NEUROSCIENCE RESEARCH PROGRESS

AMYOTROPHIC LATERAL SCLEROSIS

FROM DIAGNOSIS TO TREATMENT

Neuroscience Research Progress

Additional books and e-books in this series can be found on Nova's website under the Series tab.

NEUROSCIENCE RESEARCH PROGRESS

AMYOTROPHIC LATERAL SCLEROSIS

FROM DIAGNOSIS TO TREATMENT

JULIE SØRENSEN
EDITOR

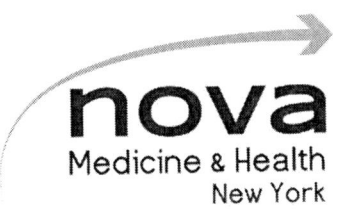

Copyright © 2020 by Nova Science Publishers, Inc.

All rights reserved. No part of this book may be reproduced, stored in a retrieval system or transmitted in any form or by any means: electronic, electrostatic, magnetic, tape, mechanical photocopying, recording or otherwise without the written permission of the Publisher.

We have partnered with Copyright Clearance Center to make it easy for you to obtain permissions to reuse content from this publication. Simply navigate to this publication's page on Nova's website and locate the "Get Permission" button below the title description. This button is linked directly to the title's permission page on copyright.com. Alternatively, you can visit copyright.com and search by title, ISBN, or ISSN.

For further questions about using the service on copyright.com, please contact:
Copyright Clearance Center
Phone: +1-(978) 750-8400 Fax: +1-(978) 750-4470 E-mail: info@copyright.com

NOTICE TO THE READER

The Publisher has taken reasonable care in the preparation of this book, but makes no expressed or implied warranty of any kind and assumes no responsibility for any errors or omissions. No liability is assumed for incidental or consequential damages in connection with or arising out of information contained in this book. The Publisher shall not be liable for any special, consequential, or exemplary damages resulting, in whole or in part, from the readers' use of, or reliance upon, this material. Any parts of this book based on government reports are so indicated and copyright is claimed for those parts to the extent applicable to compilations of such works.

Independent verification should be sought for any data, advice or recommendations contained in this book. In addition, no responsibility is assumed by the Publisher for any injury and/or damage to persons or property arising from any methods, products, instructions, ideas or otherwise contained in this publication.

This publication is designed to provide accurate and authoritative information with regard to the subject matter covered herein. It is sold with the clear understanding that the Publisher is not engaged in rendering legal or any other professional services. If legal or any other expert assistance is required, the services of a competent person should be sought. FROM A DECLARATION OF PARTICIPANTS JOINTLY ADOPTED BY A COMMITTEE OF THE AMERICAN BAR ASSOCIATION AND A COMMITTEE OF PUBLISHERS.

Additional color graphics may be available in the e-book version of this book.

Library of Congress Cataloging-in-Publication Data

Names: Sørensen, Julie, editor.
Title: Amyotrophic lateral sclerosis: from diagnosis to treatment / Julie Sørensen, editor.
Identifiers: LCCN 2020028219 (print) | LCCN 2020028220 (ebook) | ISBN 9781536181937 (paperback) | ISBN 9781536182743 (adobe pdf)
Subjects: LCSH: Amyotrophic lateral sclerosis. | Amyotrophic lateral sclerosis--Diagnosis. | Amyotrophic lateral sclerosis--Treatment.
Classification: LCC RC406.A24 A4824 2020 (print) | LCC RC406.A24 (ebook) | DDC 616.8/39--dc23
LC record available at https://lccn.loc.gov/2020028219
LC ebook record available at https://lccn.loc.gov/2020028220

Published by Nova Science Publishers, Inc. † *New York*

Contents

Preface		vii
Chapter 1	Neuroimaging in Preclinical Models of ALS *Rodolfo G. Gatto and Carina Weissmann*	1
Chapter 2	Linguistic Patterns in the Cognitive-Affective Processing of Illness Experience: A Case-Control Study of Patients with Amyotrophic Lateral Sclerosis *Andrea Caputo*	99
Chapter 3	Sensory Denervation in Motor Neuron Disease *Baris Isak*	125
Chapter 4	Non-Invasive Ventilation in ALS *Maurizia Lanza, Anna Annunziata and Giuseppe Fiorentino*	155
Index		181

PREFACE

Amyotrophic Lateral Sclerosis: From Diagnosis to Treatment focuses on two aspects of neuroimaging related to amyotrophic lateral sclerosis that have greatly evolved in the last decades: the development of optical tools in the biology field and advances in the field of magnetic resonance imaging.

Therapeutic writing and expressive disclosure interventions have been demonstrated to facilitate the emotional processing of thoughts and feelings about the amyotrophic lateral sclerosis experience, with relevant implications for illness adjustment.

Based on these premises, the authors explore the linguistic patterns in the cognitive-affective processing of illness experience in people with amyotrophic lateral sclerosis.

Following this, the authors discuss recent studies that offer a new perspective on sensory networks in motor neuron diseases to understand the true extent and patophysiology of amyotrophic lateral sclerosis and suggest new potential biomarkers for the diagnosis of this tragic disease.

The closing study focuses on the respiratory involvement of amyotrophic lateral sclerosis, which is the principal cause of death. Amyotrophic lateral sclerosis is characterized by respiratory failure consequent to respiratory muscles dysfunction, as well as bulbar muscles which support the upper airways, developing in dyspnoea and impaired sleep.

Chapter 1 - This chapter explores the expansion of imaging techniques applied to the study of preclinical models of Amyotrophic Lateral Sclerosis (ALS). The continuous development of neuroimaging techniques has been critical to advance the authors' understanding of neurodegenerative processes; and in the biological sciences, led the way to new discoveries of the molecular mechanisms of degeneration in ALS. The authors will focus on two neuroimaging aspects that have greatly evolved in the last decades related to ALS research: the development of optical tools in the biology field, and advances in the field of Magnetic Resonance Imaging (MRI). The addition of fluorescent tags in optical microscopy has been critical to study new molecular and structural markers at earlier stages of the disease. These fluorescent labels used in *in vitro* as well as *in vivo* assays, combined with improvements in computational algorithms and hardware, led to new levels of imaging analysis with higher precision. Moreover, the field of biology gained greatly from the advancements in genetics, and this allowed to partially reproduce, in animal models, the genetic mutations seen in human diseases. The proper choice of animals and imaging models to analyze molecular mechanisms of neurodegenerative diseases or test new compounds, nevertheless, remains a challenge. In parallel, technical advancements in MRI opened new possibilities within the neurosciences, giving access to intact neuraxial structures. Further, improvements in magnetic field strengths led to higher imaging resolution outputs. The authors aim this to be a cohesive overview of the available imaging research tools in ALS research and how their combination places us a step closer to finding a definitive treatment for this disease.

Chapter 2 - In recent times, narrative medicine has been developed to recognize, interpret, and make decisions from patients' experiences by focusing on illness-related psychosocial aspects, especially in chronic and rare conditions. With regard to this, research has highlighted the importance of illness stories for the improvement of perceived quality of life among people with Amyotrophic Lateral Sclerosis (ALS). Indeed, therapeutic writing and expressive disclosure interventions have been demonstrated to facilitate the emotional processing of thoughts and feelings about the ALS experience, with relevant implications for illness adjustment. Based on these premises, the current study aimed at exploring the linguistic patterns in the cognitive-affective processing of illness experience in people with ALS.

To this purpose, a case-control study was conducted on the illness stories of 12 adult Italian patients with ALS (8 women and 4 men), compared to a sample of 12 illness stories of patients (matched by gender) affected by other diverse rare diseases (anorectal atresia, Poland syndrome, and idiopathic pulmonary hypertension). The stories were retrieved through the Internet-based database of the Italian National Centre for Rare Diseases, as part of a community-based participatory project promoted by the Medical Ethics Committee of the Italian National Health Service. Several linguistic measures were inspected, referring to lexical variety (i.e., Average Word Frequency, Type-Token Ratio, and Hapax Percentage), referential activity and semantic specificities. Non-parametric Independent t-tests (Mann-Whitney U) were used to compare indexes of lexical variety and referential activity; whereas, specificity analyses were performed through T-Lab software to compare the vocabularies referring to patients with and without ALS.

The results showed no difference in lexical variety. Instead, with regard to referential activity a higher level of discrepancy between discourse organization and sensory imagery of language ($Mdn = 4$) was found in patients with ALS, compared to patients with other rare diseases ($Mdn = 1.5$), $U = 37.5, p < .05, r = .41$. Besides, some differences emerged that were close to the margin of statistical significance, indicating that narratives of participants with ALS had lower scores of clarity ($Mdn = 4.5$), $U = 39, p = .055, r = -.39$, and discourse organization ($Mdn = 11$), $U = 38.5, p = .052, r = -.40$, than their counterparts ($Mdn = 7$ and $Mdn = 13.5$, respectively). Then, specificity analyses highlighted a higher focus on disease-related impairments, a reduced contextualization of illness into one's life story, and greater efforts to restore a sense of normality in utterances of patients with ALS.

Overall, the present study suggests a biographical disruption caused by illness that threatens self-identity and the quality of symbolization function, as emerging from narratives of patients with ALS compared to those of patients affected by other rare conditions. Narrative medicine could thus benefit from such fruitful insights in order to better understand patients' perspectives, as well as to implement narrative skills in daily practice to enrich general clinical information focused on patients' needs and challenges.

Chapter 3 - Identification of amyotrophic lateral sclerosis (ALS) requires demonstration of denervation in motor fibres while sensory fibres are frequently expected to be spared. However, different aspects of sensory involvement in this disease have been extensively reported by many groups for the last three decades. Unfortunately, both the studies with conflicting results and the catastrophic clinical picture due to motor neuron degeneration placed sensory involvement in a relatively neglected position. Today, studies with a new perspective on sensory network in motor neuron diseases are conducted to understand the true extent and patophysiology of ALS and suggest new potential biomarkers to diagnose this tragic disease.

Chapter 4 - The distinctive feature of ALS is its rapid and severe development: the average survival is three years of the onset of the first symptoms and six months after the start of diaphragmatic dysfunction, in the inadequacy of treatment. Respiratory involvement of ALS is the principal cause of death. During the disease time, ALS is characterized by respiratory failure consequent to respiratory muscles dysfunction as well as bulbar muscles which support the upper airways, developing in dyspnoea and impaired sleep, with consequent severe suffering. Respiratory inability progresses gradually and leads to improved CO_2 in the blood; usually, first, at night during sleep; later, during all the day. Hypercapnia produces compromising clinical manifestations such as sleep disruptions, daytime fatigue, cognitive impairment, and depression. Since 1999 with non-invasive ventilation (NIV) has become an essential part of the treatment of ALS that significantly increases survival, quality of life and cognitive performances. From 2006 to the present time, not only has it been demonstrated that non-invasive ventilation (NIV) is challenging to adjust in this setting, but also that NIV must be integrated into multidisciplinary control, taking into description improvement of the disease and the patient's living conditions outside of the hospital. The initial NIV settings are simple, but the progression of the disease, ventilator dependence and upper airway involvement sometimes make long-term adjustment of NIV more complicated, with a significant impact on survival. Adjustment of NIV in ALS shows that correction of leaks, management of obstructive apnoea and compliance to the patient's degree of ventilator dependence improve the prognosis. Non-ventilatory factors also impact the efficacy of NIV, and various answers have been reported and must be applied, including cough assist techniques, control of excess salivation and malnutrition. More advanced use of NIV also needs pulmonologists to master the associated end-of-life palliative care, as well as the modalities of interrupting ventilation when it becomes unreasonable. ALS also impairs cough function, appearing in frequent episodes of bronchial congestion and infection. The ALS patient's family plays a principal role in supportive care and everyday management of treatment, including end-of-life palliative care. The impact on the patient's family is devastating, as a consequence of the mixed motor deficit and respiratory failure and the accelerated course of the disease, for which no therapeutic strategy is available.

In: Amyotrophic Lateral Sclerosis
Editor: Julie Sørensen

ISBN: 978-1-53618-193-7
© 2020 Nova Science Publishers, Inc.

Chapter 1

NEUROIMAGING IN PRECLINICAL MODELS OF ALS

Rodolfo G. Gatto[1,*], *MD, PhD*
and Carina Weissmann[2], *PhD*

[1]Department of Bioengineering,
University of Illinois at Chicago, Chicago, IL, US
[2]Insituto de Fisiología Biología Molecular y Neurociencias,
IFIBYNE-CONICET, University of Buenos Aires, Argentina

ABSTRACT

This chapter explores the expansion of imaging techniques applied to the study of preclinical models of Amyotrophic Lateral Sclerosis (ALS). The continuous development of neuroimaging techniques has been critical to advance our understanding of neurodegenerative processes; and in the biological sciences, led the way to new discoveries of the molecular mechanisms of degeneration in ALS. We will focus on two neuroimaging aspects that have greatly evolved in the last decades related to ALS research: the development of optical tools in the biology field, and advances in the field of Magnetic Resonance Imaging (MRI). The addition

---

* Corresponding Author's Email: rgatto@uic.edu; rodogatto@gmail.com.

of fluorescent tags in optical microscopy has been critical to study new molecular and structural markers at earlier stages of the disease. These fluorescent labels used in *in vitro* as well as *in vivo* assays, combined with improvements in computational algorithms and hardware, led to new levels of imaging analysis with higher precision. Moreover, the field of biology gained greatly from the advancements in genetics, and this allowed to partially reproduce, in animal models, the genetic mutations seen in human diseases. The proper choice of animals and imaging models to analyze molecular mechanisms of neurodegenerative diseases or test new compounds, nevertheless, remains a challenge. In parallel, technical advancements in MRI opened new possibilities within the neurosciences, giving access to intact neuraxial structures. Further, improvements in magnetic field strengths led to higher imaging resolution outputs. We aim this to be a cohesive overview of the available imaging research tools in ALS research and how their combination places us a step closer to finding a definitive treatment for this disease.

Keywords: amyotrophic lateral sclerosis, animal models, neuroimaging, optical microscopy, MRI diffusion

1. INTRODUCTION

Since its description in 1869 by the French neurologist Jean-Martin Charcot, Amyotrophic lateral sclerosis (ALS), has been described as a fatal adult onset neurodegenerative disease characterized by the selective and progressive death of both upper and lower motoneurons, leading to a progressive paralysis, respiratory depression and death generally within 2–5 years after onset. Approximately 5–10% of ALS cases are familial (fALS) with a Mendelian pattern of inheritance. The remaining 90% ALS cases are categorized as sporadic mutations (sALS). Only a fraction of fALS cases have mutations in specific genes associated, for the rest, the etiology remains unknown. Despite the actual limited advances on its treatment and prognosis, exponential improvements on imaging technologies have led to an unprecedented advance in our comprehension of the disease. As a result, the discovery of new bioimaging markers is critical to detect and monitor how genetic anomalies of this disease can be linked to early structural changes. The development of new genetic tools and improved biological models have increased our chances to accelerate the progress of new therapeutic approaches. In order to perform preclinical studies and study the etiology and the molecular mechanisms as well as design and test new therapeutic targets and molecules, several *in vitro* and *in vivo* experimental models have been stablished, that reproduce key features of the disease. In this chapter, we aim to provide the reader with an updated overview of biological models and neuroimaging techniques in ALS research.

2. PRECLINICAL MODELS OF ALS

Knowledge of the cellular and molecular pathophysiological mechanisms associated with the disease helps in the design of effective treatments. For this purpose, the use of experimental models is essential to understand how to ameliorate the damage caused by ALS. During the last decades, the principal hypotheses proposed to explain the mechanisms of neuronal degeneration have been derived mostly from *in vitro* and invertebrate models. Based on the accessibility and advances of new genomic tools, these models have provided a significant amount of information expanding our knowledge. However, while invertebrate models have yielded important insights, vertebrate models in general provide more translatable results to human disease because of their increased genetic homology. Cellular loss and phenotypical analysis are easily performed in an intact physiological organism, but the increase in complexity requires the experimenter to be aware of an increasing number of variables during the progress of the disease. Hence, the importance of simple models should not be understated, as advantageous when dissecting specific mechanisms to begin with, but the phenotypical outputs with intact organisms, conserved gene pathways and complex patterns of inheritance, makes *in vivo* model systems a necessary tool to study specific functional aspects in neurodegenerative diseases as well as for drug testing.

2.1. Cellular Systems and *In Vitro* Models in ALS

To understand mechanisms involved in ALS and identify novel therapeutic targets, a range of models are used. From biochemical systems to cell systems, the idea is to model certain aspects found in ALS and analyze it initially in a simple model. Protein misfolding -one important feature present in ALS- is described as the conversion of proteins from their normal, mostly soluble and functional three-dimensional conformation into aberrant, often insoluble, non-functional one (Liscic and Breljak 2011). This can result in a toxic gain or loss-of-function or a combination of both, which lead to neurodegeneration in the context of ALS or many other neurodegenerative diseases for that matter.

Other features that characterize ALS pathology are axonal retraction, loss of cell bodies of the upper and lower motor neurons, occurrence of astrogliosis and microgliosis, and the presence of ubiquitin-positive inclusions in surviving neurons (Saberi et al. 2015). Therefore, the analysis of the molecular pathways leading to aggregation, autophagy, RNA metabolism, and intracellular cell trafficking becomes relevant in ALS pathology. All these pathways are amenable to analysis in cell models, that lack the complexity and additional variables present in a whole organism. To study in detail the molecular events associated, several cellular models have been proposed.

This section will briefly introduce different relevant models of ALS, and in later sections, there will be examples of information obtained by using them with different imaging techniques. We subdivided these models in the following categories:

2.1.1. Cell Models in ALS

Among common cell models used in ALS research are the mouse neural hybrid cell line (MN-1), which expresses motor neuron features and high affinity glutamate transporters; the mouse motor neuron hybridoma line NSC-34, a hybridoma cell line derived from the fusion of neuroblastoma cells with mice spinal cord cells; as well as primary cells, such as the mouse primary spinal cord culture (Schlachetzki, Saliba, and Oliveira 2013). All these models allow the exogenous expression of proteins and mutations involved in the disease to analyze how this might lead to pathological mechanisms. Therefore, mutant ALS-associated proteins, such as superoxide dismutase 1 (SOD1), TAR DNA binding protein 43 (TDP-43), and fused in sarcoma (FUS) among others have been analyzed in different cell models (Moujalled et al. 2017, Gomes, Escrevente, and Costa 2010). Focusing especially on gene function or toxicity related to the overexpression of the wild type or mutant proteins. Even though cell models do not recapitulate the complexity of human disease, they provide important information on biological functions of ALS-associated genes and proteins (Van Damme, Robberecht, and Van Den Bosch 2017).

2.1.2. Yeast Models in ALS

Yeasts have been an undisputedly productive model organism for elucidating fundamental eukaryotic cellular mechanisms. Two thirds of their genome – which has been fully sequenced (Galibert et al. 1996) – have domains with significant homology to human genes; in addition this fast growing model, is cheap and easy to control (Kryndushkin and Shewmaker 2011, Robinson 2011). Approximately 500 genes implicated in human disease have a direct ortholog in yeast, thus making yeast an interesting model to study human disease. The cellular processes that involve protein misfolding -of particular importance in neurodegenerative diseases-, and in turn the cellular responses to protein misfolding, i.e., cellular stress response pathways (Heat Shock Response, the antioxidant response and the unfold response) are also highly conserved between humans and yeast (Winderickx et al. 2008). In addition, a multitude of genetic, microscopic, and biochemical tools have been developed in yeast research leading to the detection of novel genetic and protein-protein interactions.

With the expression of ALS-associated proteins, yeast models have enormously contributed to recapitulating major hallmarks of ALS pathology, including protein aggregation, mis-localization and cellular toxicity (Di Gregorio and Duennwald 2018a). Robinson highlighted the importance of yeast in ALS research with the work of two different groups: Ju et al. 2011 and Sun et al. 2011 that shed light on how defects in RNA processing and transport are among the central elements in ALS pathophysiology. Both groups analyzed FUS expression in yeast and supported the hypothesis that mis localization of the nuclear protein to the cytoplasm, rather than mutation per se is key to the disease pathogenesis (Ju et al. 2011, Robinson 2011, Sun et al. 2011). In addition, many of the complex mechanisms underlying ALS onset might be rooted in protein-protein interactions. Hence, yeasts are an optimal platform for the discovery of novel interactors but also for the characterization of those interactions as easily performed via the two hybrid system, as well as to analyse the cytotoxicity induced by ALS proteins through phenotypic screening (Suk 2017) (Figley and Gitler 2013).

2.1.3. Stem Cells in ALS

Stem cells are generally defined as cells that are capable of self-renewal and that possess the ability to differentiate into multiple types of cells (Dantuma, Merchant, and Sugaya 2010). Mesenchymal stem cells (MSCs) are multipotent adult stem cells that can be easily extracted from various adult connective tissues (i.e., bone marrow and adipose tissue) and can differentiate into a variety of cells (Marconi et al. 2013, Tang 2017). Besides their use in research, stem cell therapy using MSCs is a promising potential treatment option for ALS, given MSCs remarkable plasticity and ability to differentiate into multiple neuronal lineages. They are consequently a valuable source for replacement cell therapy (Hajivalili et al. 2016). When locally or systemically transplanted, stem cells are capable of migrating to disease-associated regions to exert the desired therapeutic effect (Mao, Zhang, and Chen 2015).Though motor neuron replacement remains as a possibility in some clinical studies to treat ALS with stem cells, there is a growing trend to use stem cells as support cells for dying motor neurons as they are already connected to the muscle (Thomsen, Gowing, Svendsen, et al. 2014). However, safety and possible clinical efficacy still require further assessment (Petrou et al. 2016). Because naturally occurring stem cells have limitations, scientists have developed a method for increasing pluripotency within non-pluripotent cells. The latter cells are termed induced pluripotent stem (iPS) cells (Dantuma, Merchant, and Sugaya 2010).

Human induced pluripotent stem cells (iPSCs) provides another opportunity to explore molecular phenotypes of ALS within human cells particularly for modeling sporadic fALS, as well as providing a personalized or targeted approach to therapy development(Fujimori et al. 2018). Moreover additional glial cell lines can be generated, adding a more comprehensive insight into this pathology (Birger et al. 2019). More importantly, iPSC-derived neurons may reveal salient early-stage disease-driving mechanisms that constitute more potent targets than those identified through end-stage post-mortem tissue sample analyses. Thus, a combination of non-human and human iPSC models, confirmed by ALS genetic or post-mortem studies, may yield the most benefit in identifying robust disease mechanisms and promising clinical compounds (Hawrot, Imhof, and Wainger 2020). Nevertheless, the acquisition of mutations that may be acquired during reprogramming or subsequent passaging of iPSC has been recognized as a potential complicating factor to this technology (Richard and Maragakis 2015). The advent of induced-pluripotent stem cells and three-dimensional cell culture provide tools that are revolutionizing the study of human diseases by permitting analysis of patient-derived human tissue with non-invasive procedures. As such, brain organoids, self-organizing neural structures that can mimic human fetal brain development, have now been harnessed to develop alternative models and could represent a game change for the *in vitro* study of neurodegenerative diseases such as ALS (Grenier, Kao, and Diamandis 2020).

2.2. Invertebrate Transgenics Models of ALS

The use of invertebrate animals is another practical tool in ALS research. They add another layer of complexity that cell models lack: the interplay that occurs between neurons and their surrounding environment in a living organism to help identify the genetic networks in neurodegeneration.

2.2.1. Worm Models

Due to their availability and exponential growth, worms such as *Caenorhabditis elegans* can be genetically manipulated in the pan-neuronal expression of proteins. About 35% of human genes have a functional orthologue in worms, whose nervous system is simple and well characterized (Van Damme, Robberecht, and Van Den Bosch 2017). The generation of worm lines carrying a single-copy knock-in of the mutant version of human protein super oxide dismutase (SOD1), led to interesting findings, as a model that avoids over expression of the SOD1 and thus, makes it possible to analyze gain as well as loss of toxic function associated to SOD1 mutation in different neurons (Baskoylu et al. 2018). In this model, SOD1 alterations produced a locomotor defect associated with synaptic dysfunction, possibly involving deficient trafficking of pre-synaptic vesicles and muscular dysfunction(Wang et al. 2009); a mechanism that has also been attributed in other studies to a SOD1 G85R mutant (Ogawa et al. 2015, Baskoylu et al. 2018).

Mutations in other genes, like the *C9orf72* were also analyzed in worms. Discovered approximately a decade ago, the GGGGCC hexanucleotide repeat expansion (HRE) in the *C9orf72* gene is recognized as the most common genetic cause of ALS and frontotemporal dementia (FTD) (Hayes and Rothstein 2016). Therefore many studies have used worms as models amenable to phenotypically reproduce the mutant forms of *C9orf72* (Therrien et al. 2013), as well as FUS (Murakami et al. 2012) and TDP-43 proteinopathy (Ash et al. 2010, Liachko, Guthrie, and Kraemer 2010) to test potential therapeutic compounds which could potentially ameliorate the progression of the disease (Jiang et al. 2014, Ikenaka et al. 2019).

2.2.2. Fly Models

Drosophila melanogaster, commonly known as the fruit fly, has been one of the most influential models in genetics research and disease modeling (Casci and Pandey 2015). 75% of human genes have a functional orthologue in flies. Their nervous system are also quite sophisticated with 100,000 neurons (Van Damme, Robberecht, and Van Den Bosch 2017). Interestingly, this model has contributed to several findings in ALS and novel aspects have been discovered by analyzing ALS transgenic flies. Particularly, human SOD1 mutations in a *Drosophila* knock-in reveals similar dosage-sensitive gain-and-loss-of-function components in a phenotype exhibiting neurodegeneration, locomotor deficits, and shortened life span (Sahin et al. 2017). Moreover, as mutations in genes that regulate RNA metabolism are a major cause of inherited ALS, the study of these genes in the *Drosophila* nervous system has identifyied key pathways contributing to nucleo-cytoplasmic transport and stress granule assembly (Zhang, Coyne, and Lloyd 2018). In addition, a novel aspect that has been analyzed in this model is the retrotransposon-like element (RTE). RTEs are genomic parasite selfish genetic elements that are coded within our genomes that use an RNA intermediate retrotranscribed by a reverse transcriptase into cDNA copy; and this cDNA is inserted into a new genomic location at the site of double stranded DNA breaks created by an endonuclease activity encoded by the RTE. Krug et al. worked on the hypothesis that a loss of control of RTEs contributes to the cumulative degeneration observed with TDP-43 protein aggregation pathology that is observed in a variety of neurodegenerative disorders, including ALS and FTLD. They proposed that this loss of control of RTEs is the result of the negative impact of TDP-43 pathology on general RTE suppression mechanisms that are most prevalently relied upon in somatic tissue such as the brain. Increased RTE activity occurs in the brain during aging and expression of RTEs has been detected in neurodegenerative diseases, as in cortical tissue of ALS patients. To test whether RTEs play a role in TDP-43 mediated neurodegeneration, an established *Drosophila* transgenic model was used to examine whether RTE activation causally contributes to TDP-43 mediated toxicity and cell death. Although the versatility of *Drosophila* has been demonstrated in ALS research using FUS (Steyaert et al. 2018), C9oRF7, (Cunningham et al. 2019, Kokona et al. 2019) and TDP-43, (Krug et al. 2017) transgenic models, this model has limitations mostly based on differences in certain molecular pathways and degrees of brain connectome complexity, thus, the extrapolation of results into the human population is difficult. Nonetheless, most of the Drosophila knock-in models, as described, captures important aspects of human ALS phenotypes and provides a powerful and a proven useful tool for further genetic studies (Hirth 2010, Bilen and Bonini 2005) that pave the way to further analysis.

2.3. Vertebrate Transgenic Models of ALS

As described in the previous sections, invertebrate models have been of paramount help to analyze different mutations in ALS. These model organisms have highly malleable genomes allowing for a rapid generation of transgenic lines to provide insight on gene functions and protein network interactions. In addition, certain pathways can be analyzed without any other confounding variables that exist in organisms of higher complexity. In that regard, they constitute an excellent first step in research that open the way to further testing and analysis in vertebrate models. In turn, vertebrate models represent a higher degree of complexity and show a greater sequence conservation with human genome, and thus, can model more closely human diseases (Tovar, Santa-Cruz, and Tapia 2009, Alrafiah 2018). In the case of ALS, which derives its name from its neuropathological hallmark: the degeneration of motor neurons in the spinal anterior horn and motor cortex and loss of axons in the lateral columns of the spinal cord; vertebrate models, provides researchers with a spinal cord to model with (Saberi et al. 2015). In the following sections we will introduce different vertebrate models that are used in ALS research.

2.3.1. Fish Models

Transgenic zebra fish *(Danio rerio)* lines have been used to investigate different ALS-related mutations. In the original ALS zebrafish SOD1 mutated models, not only did these develop early motor axonopathy (Lemmens et al. 2007, Ramesh et al. 2010) and neuromuscular effects (Sakowski et al. 2012), but also early interneuron dysfunction (McGown et al. 2013). Other mutations that have been analyzed in these models are those present in TDP-43, like the G348C mutation (identified in around 5% of familiar and 1% of sporadic ALS cases). The lack of effect in the function of this gene, could point to a toxic gain-of-function. In a study by Ciuria et al. the expression of the mutant but not the wild-type human TDP-43 in zebrafish embryos induced a reduction of locomotor activity in response to touch as well as a moderate axonopathy of the motor neurons of the spinal cord, with premature branching (Lissouba et al. 2018) and neuromuscular junction abnormalities (Bose, Armstrong, and Drapeau 2019).

Studies using zebrafish to analize the hexanucleotide repeat expansion in the *(C9orf72)* gene also showed that a loss of function of C9orf72 causes motor deficits (Shaw et al. 2018, Ciura et al. 2013).

A study using a knockdown zebrafish model of FUS showed impaired motor activity and reduced neuro-muscular junction (NMJ) and demonstred that FUS loss results in a defect of presynaptic function (Armstrong and Drapeau 2013).

2.3.2. Rodent Models

Among the advantages in using rodent models, are their high degree of genetic homology to humans, thus great relevance to human physiology, and the possibility to study early genetic, neuropathological and phenotypical abnormalities proven to be related to the human disease (Durand et al. 2006, de Oliveira, Alves, and Chadi 2013, Fogarty, Mu, et al. 2016, Fogarty, Noakes, and Bellingham 2015). Based on their low cost, scalability and reproducibility, murine models *(Mus musculus)* are the most common mammalian models used in the study of ALS (Table 1). The first breakthrough in the development of rodent models to study ALS came with the discovery, in the early 90s, that mutations in the gene encoding SOD1 were related to the disease and this mutation was introduced in a mouse model (Gurney 1994).

The G93A-SOD1 mutation was the first one introduced in transgenic mice; later on, other SOD1 mutations led to the production of more lines, and the use of different promoters (Mina, Konsolaki, and Zagoraiou 2018). However, the G93A-SOD1 mice remains the most widely used, since it shows selective vulnerability of motor neurons as described in the human disease. Muscle fibers become denervated, axons degenerate, and spinal

Table 1. Most common murine models used in ALS research

Murine Model	Genetic Anomaly and Mutation	Phenotype	Key References
Murine Models of Spontaneous Forms of ALS (sALS)			
Wobbler (Vps54)	A point mutation in Vps54, component of the GARP vesicle-tethering involved in the retrograde vesicle transport from endosomes.	Muscle atrophy, astrogliosis, microgliosis, hyperexcitability, mitochondrial dysfunction, axonal transport defects, neurofilament aggregation, and ubiquitin-positive protein aggregation.	Moser et al. (2013) Schmitt-John et al. (2015)
BSSG exposure	Chronic exposure to dietary sterol glucosides.	Progressive motor dysfunction persists after BSSG exposure has been discontinued; loss of motor neurons; reduced NMJ integrity; astrocytosis; evidence of microgliosis; neuronal cell death in pathologically relevant regions.	Wilson et al. (2002) Tabata et al. (2008)
Murine Models of Familiar Forms of ALS (fALS)			
G93A-SOD1	Mutations in the Cu/Zn superoxide dismutase 1 (SOD1) gene. More than 160 missense mutations in the SOD1 gene have been found to be linked to ALS. Transgenic mice of more than 13 different SOD1 mutant variants are available.	Progressive motor dysfunction: loss of motor neurons: axonal denervation; impaired NMJ integrity; proteinopathy; mitochondrial dysfunction; glutamate mediated excitotoxicity; axonal transport defects; microgliosis; astrocytosis; impaired glial function; T cell invasion; premature death. Changes in dendritic structure and spine density on vulnerable cortical pyramidal neurons.	Gerney et al. (1994) Nardo et al. (2016) Fogarty et al. (2016)
TDP-43-Q331K	Mutation gene encoding for TAR DNA-binding protein (TARDBP or TDP-43).	Progressive motor dysfunction; cortical and spinal motor neuron dendritic synaptic abnormalities; motor neuron and axon degeneration; reduced integrity of NMJ; muscle atrophy, astrocytosis and microglia infiltration; defects in RNA processing, neuronal death.	Igaz et al. (2011) Tsao et al. (2012) Fogarty et al. (2016) Arnold et al. (2016) Huang et al. (2020)

Murine Model	Genetic Anomaly and Mutation	Phenotype	Key References
		Murine Models of Familiar Forms of ALS (fALS)	
C9orf72	Expansion of a hexanucleotide (GGGGCC) repeat in chromosome 9 open reading frame 72 (C9orf72). Presence of greater than 30 repeats is considered pathogenic.	Paralysis, motor neuron loss; Neurite density loss; Reduced NMJ integrity; accumulation of antisense RNA foci; DPR and TPD-43 aggregation, reduced lifespan	Liu Y et al. (2016) Hayes et al. (2016) Batra et al. (2019)
FUS	Mutations in the Fused-in-Sarcoma (FUS) gene encoding a 526 amino-acid RNA-binding protein. Over-expressing human WT FUS (hFUS +/+) or Human aggregate prone FUS-variant lacking Nuclear localization signal and RNA binding motif.	Full KO does not have evident phenotype. Mutations expressing lower level than endogenous fuss present with severe motor disfunction; FUS positive inclusion in LMN and ubiquitinated inclusions; Significant SC neuronal loos and neuroinflammation	Mitchel et al. (2013) Shelkovnikova et al. (2013)
TBK1	Heterozygous loss-of-function; mutations of TANK-binding kinase 1 (TBK1)	Homozygous KO of Tbk1 is embryonically lethal. Cognitive and locomotor deficits.; neurofibrillary tangles; abnormal dendrites and reduced dendrite spine density; loss of cortical synapses; p62 and ubiquitin-positive aggregates; impaired autophagy mechanisms	Brenner et al. (2019) Duan et al. (2019)

Abbreviations: GARP, Golgi-associated retrograde protein; BSSG, beta-sitosterol beta-D: -glucoside; NMJ, neuromuscular junction; sALS, spontaneous form of ALS; fALS, familiar form of ALS; KO, knock-out mouse, WT, wild type.

motor neurons undergo cell death. In this model, various pathological changes and mechanisms have been described including mitochondrial abnormalities, oxidative stress, glutamatergic toxicity, cytoskeletal dysfunction, defective axonal transport, and repeated denervation and reinnervation of neuromuscular junctions. In addition, via the expression of mutant SOD1 in astrocytes and microglia, these cells were recognized as an important driving force in the disease progression (Mead et al. 2011).

Despite the advantages of this model, variability both in the onset and the progression of the disease in different strains exists. Transgenic SOD1 rodent models have fluctuating ages of disease onset and disease progression

(Haulcomb et al. 2015). Moreover, the development of ALS-like symptoms in these mice are now known to be largely dependent upon factors such as: SOD1 mutation; transgene expression level; gender and genetic background (Philips and Rothstein 2015, Heiman-Patterson et al. 2005, Mancuso et al. 2012, de Oliveira, Alves, and Chadi 2013). The two most widely used strains, C56BL/6 (B6) and B6SJL, show differences in the onset of motor neuron abnormalities, appearing later in B6SJL mice, but progressing more rapidly. Moreover, mean survival in the B6 background is significantly higher, and in contrast to the B6/SJL and SJL backgrounds, there are no differences in survival between males and females. These phenotypic differences could not be explained by alterations in copy number, but were traced back to the difference in the strains, and became the first report of a shortened lifespan when the G93A-SOD1 transgene is placed on the SJL/J background, and an increased survival with no gender influence when the transgene is placed on the C57BL/6J background (Heiman-Patterson et al. 2005). The commonly used SOD1 strain is maintained by crossing C57BL66SJL hemizygous male transgenic mice with female C57BL66SJL/J hybrids; this leads to genetic variation. To avoid this "noise", studies like the one of Mead et al. use the well-defined inbred mouse strains G93A-SOD1 transgenic mice on an inbred C57BL/6 genetic background to minimize genetic variation. All this information points to the fact that the characteristics of the strain should be taken into account in the experimental design of therapeutic studies since the potential efficacy of any new therapeutic approach is directly related with the onset of the treatment and, ultimately, with the disease progression in a specific animal model.

So far, most studies in humans have been unable to replicate any of the published positive effects of compounds in this model. This "inconsistency" has been largely attributed to "biological noise" with a poor study design in the majority of published positive neuroprotective studies; and led to recommendations for the conduct of pre-clinical studies which includes the use of litter matched controls, treatment groups and gene copy number analysis for all mice on therapeutic trials (Mead et al. 2011). Nevertheless, although many effective drugs in SOD1 mice have not been proven beneficial, or are even toxic for patients, and even if new studies challenge the validity of some of these drugs showing no significant benefit on lifespan in ALS mouse models previously tested, we should keep in mind that the only two FDA approved drugs for ALS treatment, Riluzole and Edaravone, were initially validated in SOD1 mice (Hogg et al. 2018).

Over time, new genetic mutations discovered in ALS have been incorporated in different murine models demonstrating different aspects of the mechanisms observed in ALS patients. After all, the SOD1 mouse reproduce many symptoms, but has not been able to recapitulate some features related to ALS, such as changes in RNA metabolism. Therefore, other mice transgenic lines were generated incorporating different ALS associated proteins.

Mice transgenic lines with mutations in TDP-43 provided information on other mechanisms related to ALS. TDP-43 is normally localized in the nucleus, and is associated to the regulation of gene expression; however, in the TDP-43 transgenic mice, pathological cytoplasmic aggregates associated with depletion of the nuclear protein have been described, leading to neuronal death and degeneration (Igaz et al. 2011). Using high resolution imaging, researchers have also reported increased excitatory synaptic inputs and dendritic spine densities in early stages, demonstrating substantial alterations in the motor cortex neural network, long before any degenerative phenotype could be observed (Fogarty, Klenowski, et al. 2016). Subsequently, as the mice aged, a selective cellular population vulnerability to the expression of human TDP-43 was documented (van Hummel et al. 2018). Additional studies have shown that TDP-43 protein is also expressed and distributed in the cytoplasm of oligodendrocyte cells of the spinal cord gray matter suggesting the involvement of multiple cell populations in the mechanism of this disease (Lu et al. 2016). Apart from the TDP-43 transgenic lines, the TDP-43 knock out was also informative, showing that the mouse was not viable and thus, pointing to developmental functions associated to the gene. However, none of the TDP43 transgenic models appear to develop enough ALS features, indicating that abnormal TDP43 in mice may not be enough for complete recapitulation of the disease (Gendron and Petrucelli 2011, Tsao et al. 2012).

Even though structural and functional similarities between TDP-43 and FUS exist, these proteins are differently post-translationally modified. TDP-43, for example is extensively phosphorylated and cleaved to produce toxic, aggregate prone C-terminal fragments, while endogenous FUS is maintained at full length, even during the disease (Nolan, Talbot, and Ansorge 2016). In the case of the FUS knock out mice, these displayed a reduced body weight, but no alteration in the motor phenotype, or numbers of choline-acetyltransferase positive neurons. This suggests that FUS depletion alone is insufficient to cause ALS symptoms or pathology (Kino et al. 2015). Lines overexpressing the human wild type or mutant FUS have shown, in some cases, a decline in motor functions without any cytoplasmic inclusions, with the mutant being more pathogenic than the wild type (wt) counterpart. Hence, reproducing both, the motor dysfunction phenotype, and the distinct neuropathological features of FUS-linked ALS has proven challenging in rodents. This might be explained by the methodology used to generate the mice, to an over expressing system, and might be ameliorated with the use of a BAC system (Nolan, Talbot, and Ansorge 2016).

Different mouse models were generated via introduction of different number of the hexa-repeat in the *C9orf72* gene. Transgenic mice carrying 500 repeats developed many of the neuropathological hallmarks of the disease, such as severe motor neuron degeneration and paralysis, as well as cognitive symptoms (Batra and Lee 2017, Hayes and Rothstein 2016, Liu et al. 2016).

Recently, genetic insufficiency of the protein TANK-binding kinase 1 (TBK1) has been shown to be related to ALS. The conditional neuronal deletion of TBK1 leads to cognitive and locomotor deficits in mice as well as neurofibrillary tangles, abnormal dendrites, reduced dendritic spine density, and cortical synapse loss (Duan et al. 2019). Based on the research by Brenner et al. part of the proposed mechanism of TBK1 at early and late stages are coupled to complex mechanisms of autophagia in motor neurons as well as neuroinflammation and protein dysregulation (Brenner et al. 2019). As part of the neuropathological findings, the presence of protein and RNA aggregates in the cytoplasm of motor neurons were key features present in the TBK1 mouse. The various roles of TBK1 in autophagy, especially phosphorylating adaptor proteins, suggests that this may also be an important process contributed by TBK1 mutations. Importantly, p62, OPTN, and another autophagy adaptor protein, NDP52 are all regulated by TBK1 phosphorylation, and thus, enhance the ability to link LC3-II and ubiquitinated cargo simultanously. The fact that TBK1 expression is high in neurons that are then lost during ALS suggest that loss of function in TBK1 mutations may have a greater effect in these cells (Oakes, Davies, and Collins 2017).

As previously mentioned, most ALS cases derive from spontaneous gene mutations. In mice, a mutation arose spontaneously in a C57BL/Fa strain characterized by motor neuron degeneration, this was named the wobbler mouse. The mutation, a recessive point mutation, affects the protein Vps54, a component of the Golgi-associated retrograde (GARP) complex that affects retrograde vesicle transport, i.e., the vesicle transport from endosomes to the TGN, (Moser, Bigini, and Schmitt-John 2013) leading to defects in Golgi morphology and function (Schmitt-John 2015). This mouse closely resembles human forms of sALS regarding motor neuron degeneration, muscle atrophy, reactive gliosis as well as other cellular effects like ubiquitinated protein aggregation, oxidative stress, cortical hyperexcitability and cellular transport defects. Other mouse models used in ALS are generated through the chronic administration of specific sterol glucosides diets to generate neuropathological and behavioral phenotypes resembling sALS (Tabata et al. 2008, Wilson et al. 2002).

Transgenic rat models (*Rattus norvergicus*) have also proven useful in identifying early disease progression (Thonhoff et al. 2007). Experiments in which the SOD1 mutation is overexpressed, recapitulated a significant number of the hallmark signs seen in patients with ALS. Specifically, spinal motor neuron loss occurred before degeneration of ventral root axons and denervation of NMJs. However, the knockdown of the SOD1 mutation resulted in a significant delay of disease onset, expansion of lifespan, enhanced survival of spinal motor neurons, and maintenance of NMJ (Thomsen, Gowing, Latter, et al. 2014). Thomsen et al. showed the critical role of upper motor neurons on disease onset and lifespan via targeted silencing of SOD1 in a presymptomatic G93A-SOD1 rat model in the motor cortex (Thomsen, Gowing, Latter, et al. 2014).

In regard to TDP-43 and FUS ribonucleoproteins, these are constantly expressed at substantial levels in the central nervous system throughout a rodent's lifetime playing an important role in development (Huang, Xia, and Zhou 2010). Hence, a constant and robust expression of the genes in motor neurons may render the neurons vulnerable to pathogenic mutation on these genes (Zhou et al. 2010). Apart from motoneurons, the selective expression of mutant TDP-43 in astrocytes leads to self and microglia activation, causing a progressive loss of motor neurons and the denervation and atrophy of skeletal muscles, resulting in progressive paralysis. Overall, this mechanism involves the deficiency in neuroprotective genes and induction of neurotoxic genes in glial cells (Tong et al. 2013). In terms of FUS expression in transgenic rats, as described in mice, the overexpression of a mutant human FUS has been shown to induce progressive paralysis, resembling symptoms described in ALS. FUS transgenic rats developed progressive paralysis secondary to degeneration of motor axons and displayed a substantial loss of neurons in the cortex and hippocampus accompanied by glial reaction. These results again, as in mice, suggested that mutant FUS is more toxic than the wild type to neurons and enough to induce neuronal death (Huang et al. 2011).

2.3.3. Canine Models

Development of effective treatments for ALS would be facilitated by identification of early events in the pathological cascade of disease progression in larger animals under the premise of their genetic proximity to humans. Canine (*Canis lupus*) degenerative myelopathy (CDM), an inherently striking disease on a specific breed of dogs, is comparable to some forms of ALS associated with SOD1 mutations. Compared with the SOD1 rodent models, dogs with CDM are more similar to humans in size, in the structure and complexity of their nervous systems, as well as in the duration of the disease; and since there is no genetic manipulation, it is unlikely that they possess the very high levels of mutant SOD1 expression which occur in many of the mice models. Thus, CDM seems to be a good model for the human disease (Katz et al. 2017). CDM presents similar clinical signs, neuropathological findings, and presence of mutations in the SOD1 gene; microscopic detection of axonal degeneration, demyelination and astroglia proliferation have also been described (Nardone et al. 2016). Specifically, only two SOD1 mutations have been described in CDM affected dogs (Ogawa et al. 2014, Kobatake et al. 2017, Draper et al. 2020). However, contrary to ALS, CDM neuropathology seems to involve primarily the ascending and descending tracts, indicating that the lower motor neurons remain morphologically intact even in DM affected dogs with relatively advanced clinical signs. Interestingly, acetylcholine receptor complexes in the canine muscle are intact in CDM prior to functional impairment, thus suggesting that muscle atrophy in CDM does not result from physical denervation (Katz et al. 2017). Nonetheless, this model offers a better understanding of the factors that determine the disease progression and may be beneficial for the development of effective treatments for ALS (Nardone et al. 2016).

2.3.4. Porcine Models

Transgenic pigs (*Sus scrofia*) expressing mutations in the human *SOD1 gene* have been generated and show hind limb motor defects consequence of the motor neuron degeneration which occurs in a dose- and age-dependent manner. Interestingly, in this model, mutant human SOD1 did not form cytoplasmic inclusions as in patients with ALS, but showed nuclear accumulation and ubiquitinated nuclear aggregates as those present in some ALS patient brains (Yang et al. 2014). Additional observations in this model have proved an increase in motor neuron degeneration, severe myopathy as well as TDP-43 increase as observed in humans (Crociara et al. 2019). Histological inspection of the spinal cords showed that motor neurons had shrunk and died away, followed by microgliosis and astrogliosis. SOD1-positive inclusions had settled into both spinal cord and brainstem. At the end stage of the disease, neuromuscular junctions in leg muscles were denervated. However, necrosis and inflammation had taken hold of skeletal muscles towards the end of the disease, two signs not typically seen in people with ALS. Thus, this animal model has a phenotype that recapitulates some features of human ALS, though other mechanisms are also present which do not relate to ALS. The development of transgenic swine models, however, open the opportunity to investigate ALS biomarkers within a long period before disease onset (Chieppa et al. 2014, Holm, Alstrup, and Luo 2016, Dolezalova et al. 2014).

2.3.5. Primate Models

Considering the genetic resemblance between monkeys and humans, despite the cost, some studies were carried out using this model. As an example, a study was conducted to overexpress wild-type TDP-43 in spinal cords of cynomolgus monkeys (*Macaca fascicularis*) by stereotaxic injection of an adeno-associated virus vector into the cervical cord, and examined the phenotype using behavioral, electrophysiological, neuropathological, and biochemical analyses comparing this to rodents. While rat models expressed TDP-43 only in the nucleus of motoneurons, monkeys showed regional cytoplasmic TDP-43 mislocalization with loss of nuclear TDP-43 staining in the lateral nuclear group of spinal cord innervating distal hand muscles. The study showed a species difference, with the monkey model recapitulating TDP-43 pathology in ALS to a greater extent than rodent models (Uchida et al. 2012). Recent studies have also shown that, an adeno-associated virus (AAV) encoding an artificial microRNA (miRNA) to silence expression of the *SOD1* gene can be delivered to the spinal cord of non-human primates (marmoset and macaque), and thus, the potential of using rAAVrh10 for intrathecal delivery of an miRNA as well as the feasibility of moving to animals larger than ALS mice or rats (Borel et al. 2016, Borel et al. 2018).

The induction of protein aggregates in motor neurons and microglial activation can be also induced in the Vervet monkey (*Chlorocebus Sabaeus*) by the administration of cyanotoxin β-N-methylamino-l-alanine (BMAA). The spinal cords of BMAA-fed monkeys had numerous features comparable to ALS. For instance, there were significantly fewer motor neurons, and those that were present were smaller, indicative of motor nerve cell death. Motor neurons were also found to contain Bunina bodies, characteristic formations observed in ALS (Okamoto, Mizuno, and Fujita 2008).

Aggregates containing the ALS-associated proteins TDP-43 and reactive astrogliosis and activated microglia as well as damage to myelinated axons in the lateral corticospinal tracts were also visualized (Davis et al. 2020). Altogether, such neuropathological findings suggest that primate models may serve as a useful experimental model for testing novel therapeutics for the treatment of ALS.

Biological models are continuously improving and playing an important role in understanding the mechanism of the disease as well as in the design of new therapies for ALS. Considering all the models discussed in this section, it seems clear that their biological characteristics makes some of them more suitable for specific aspects of preclinical ALS research. Logically, complex and multifactorial pathophysiology of human neurodegenerative diseases can be captured only partially through standard animal models; some are less prone to exhibit neurodegeneration-like changes (Burns et al. 2015, Morrice, Gregory-Evans, and Shaw 2018). Moreover, considering the poor track record of mouse-based translational therapies for neurodegeneration, a growing concern has been raised towards the validity of such models (Ransohoff 2018). Possibly a cross-model approach in which novel disease mechanism are identified in less complex systems and later validated in more complex ones might yield better results to translate to the clinic (Van Damme, Robberecht, and Van Den Bosch 2017). Nonetheless, part of the scientific process towards the development of new imaging methods and potential therapeutics is to critically evaluate and improve animal models of human disease assuring they are properly used. We focus our analysis in the field of ALS research.

3. OPTICAL MICROSCOPY IN ALS

The last decade has witnessed an enormous growth in the use of optical microscopy at the micron and submicron level in Neurosciences (Davidson and Abramowitz 2002). Moreover, the rapid development of new fluorescent labels has accelerated the expansion of fluorescence microscopy in the laboratory and diverse neurobiological scenarios (Figure 1). In neurodegenerative diseases, it is key to study and follow precisely all the spatiotemporal morphological alterations, which occur during the various degenerative processes continuously, resulting in neuronal death and in serious degradation of the neuronal networks (Baloyannis 2015a). Thus, the neuropathological molecular signature common to almost all sporadic ALS and most familial ALS are observed and described using different microscopy techniques. Evidently, microscopy techniques have been and still are fundamental to describe and gain insight into this as well as other diseases. Different advances in microscopy techniques used in ALS research can be mentioned, such as high resolution, multiplex and real-time imaging with good image quality, and the capability of tracking of various labeled cell types. However, there are also limitations, including the required surgical window, smaller field of view, and limited tissue penetration.

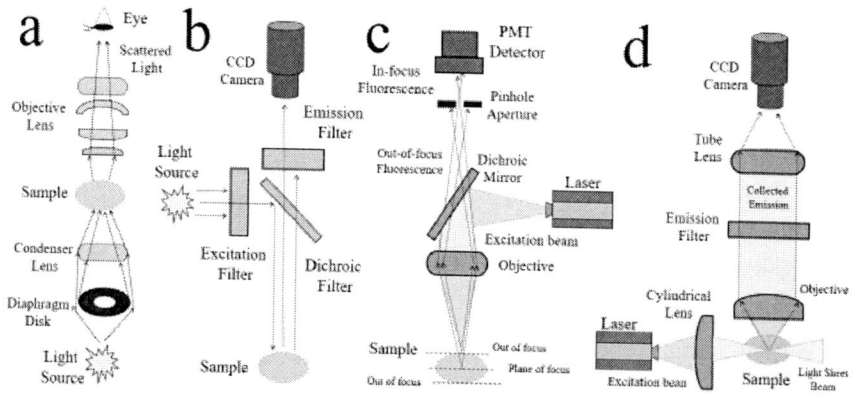

Figure 1. Diagram showing different optical microscopy modalities used in preclinical models of ALS. a - Scheme of the components in bright field microscopy. b - Fluorescence microscopy setup. c - Confocal fluorescence microscopy. d - Light sheet optical microscopy system.
Abbreviations: PMT, photon multiplier; CCD, Charged Coupled Device.

We will describe here, some of the key optical microscopy techniques instrumental for the precise visualization and estimation of the morphological alterations of neurons and neuronal circuits, enabling the study of degenerating axons, dendrites, spines, synaptic boutons and axonal terminals (Davidson and Abramowitz 2002).

3.1. Traditional Microscopy Staining Methods

Staining is used to highlight important features of the tissue as well as to enhance the tissue contrast. In this section we will mention different staining methods and markers that are most used in ALS studies.

Hematoxylin and eosin (H&E) staining is a very common and traditional method used in ALS neuropathology. Hematoxylin is a basic dye that stains the nuclei giving it a bluish color, while eosin (an acidophilic stain dye used in histology as a counter stain to hematoxylin) stains the cell's cytoplasm giving it a pinkish stain. Axons and dendrites cannot be distinguished unless there are swelling-related changes (Alturkistani, Tashkandi, and Mohammedsaleh 2015). Using Cresyl violet, neuronal Nissl bodies (the rough endoplasmic reticulum) are stained purple. Another stain commonly used for cell bodies is Toluidine blue (also known as Tolonium Chloride). This is an acidophilic metachromatic dye that selectively stains acidic tissue components (sulfates, carboxylates, and phosphate radicals). Toluidine blue (TB) has an affinity for nucleic acids, and therefore binds to nuclear material of tissues with a high DNA and RNA content (Sridharan and Shankar 2012).

The previous mentioned staining methods label neuron cell bodies but are not neuron specific. The silver staining method was introduced in histology by Camillo Golgi (black reaction) and is based on the gradual impregnation of nerve cells and their processes by silver chromate, which gives them a deep dark, almost black appearance, on a yellow background. This provides a clear insight into the morphological profile and the morphometric characteristic of brain cells (Baloyannis 2015b). During the last years, the Golgi technique has undergone a significant amount of modifications, enhancements and refinements to attain the maximal visualization of neurons (Baloyannis 2015a). Another common staining method used in disease reaserch is labeling apoptotic cells with the TUNEL staining. TUNEL stands for terminal deoxynucleotidyl transferase-mediated dUTP nick-end labeling. The TUNEL assay fluorescently labels nicked ends of fragmented DNA, thus detecting apoptosis via fluorescence microscopy due to the fluorescent reagent used (Kyrylkova et al. 2012). Another commonly staining used in ALS is the ATP stain. Fiber typing is done on recognition of distinct myosin isoforms based on their sensitivity of their ATPase activity to acid and alkaline solutions. When a muscle is incubated in a solution of pH 10.6 before the myosin ATPase reaction is performed, only predominantly fast myosin fibers will react (type II); when incubated at pH 4.3 only the fibers containing the slow myosin react (slow Type I fiber) (Stoward and Ploem 1982).

Overall, these techniques allow a clear insight into the morphological profile and the morphometric characteristics of the dendritic arbor, the dendritic branches, the spines and the estimation of the spine density as well as the morphological alterations of these elements, which are the smallest, most sensitive and vulnerable morphological part of the neuron (Baloyannis 2015b, a).

3.2. Fluorescent Microscopy Labels

3.2.1. Endogenously Expressed Fluorescent Proteins

In the animal kingdom, fluorescence proteins (FP) have evolved for visual communication purposes (Chudakov et al. 2010). The natural diversity of FPs has provided scientists with a rich palette of variants with different biochemical and spectral characteristics, which represent a huge source of potentially powerful molecular tools for several applications in the study of complex biological systems (Chen, Truong, and Ai 2017, Jensen 2012). Specifically, FPs absorb light photons at a wavelength specific to the FP, which then excites electrons to a higher energy state. As the electrons return to the ground state, energy is released as light at a different wavelength generating a color on the visible spectrum. A point of consideration using FP is their photostability, which is one of the cornerstones of a successful imaging experiment and becomes the key factor in long time series, when gathering a weak fluorescent signal (Miyawaki, Sawano, and Kogure 2003, Kremers et al. 2011). Cloning a gene of interest in frame with an FP results in a genetic construct that can be introduced into cells and organisms to highlight localization of the expressed protein of interest (Crivat and Taraska 2012, Wang, Luo, and Small 1994).

3.2.2. Fluorescence Immunohistochemistry (IHC) and Immuno-Cytological Staining

This method is used to visualize the expression of proteins and other biomolecules. IHC and ICC depend on antibodies to recognize and bind specific proteins (antigens) to help visualize dendrites, axons, synapses, neuronal nuclei, glia and so on. Either the antibody is conjugated to a fluorescent label or chromogenic enzyme, or else, a secondary antibody raised against the species of the primary is (Carter and Shieh 2010). Today, protein labeling is one of the most popular applications of FPs for visualizing protein expression, localization, translocation in living organisms, particularly in live-cell imaging (Weissmann and Brandt 2008, Gauthier-Kemper et al. 2012, Weissmann et al. 2013). In addition to protein labeling, RNA can also be visualized; in-situ hybridization is used to visualize the expression of nuclear acids, usually mRNA, and thus, determine when and where a specific gene is expressed. To perform it, a complementary sequence to the mRNA of interest as single-stranded nucleic acid probe must be generated and tagged. When the tag is fluorescent, the technique is termed FISH (Carter and Shieh 2015).

3.2.3. Fluorescent Tracers and Nanoparticles

The fundamental purpose of neuronal tracing is to visualize anatomical connections within the nervous system (Chadwick, Mc, and Nairn 1958). There is currently a significant number of fluorescent tracers available with different absorption spectra, thus permitting simultaneous labelling with multiple markers (Kobbert et al. 2000). The usefulness of these probes is overwhelming as neuroanatomical tools: the identification of retrograde axonal transport allows documentation of the cells of origin of afferent nerve fibers to a target zone. In this case, the tracer material is applied to a fiber tract or a terminal field of innervation and becomes incorporated into the cell axon and the tracer is carried back to the cell body. In the case of anterograde transport, the uptake mechanisms involve the cell soma and/or its dendrites, and the tracer material is transported along the axonal microtubular system to the cell's synaptic terminals. Fluorescent dyes are probably the most frequently used as neuroanatomical tracers representing a very useful tool in neuroscience, because labelled cells can be studied in the living material with the possibility to perform parallel experiments on the same tissue (Lu et al. 2001). Fluorescent nanoparticles have also lately found their way to studies in neurobiology (Pathak et al. 2006, Rosenthal et al. 2011, Silva 2009). Thus, the use of quantum dots has been proven valuable as nanoprobes, with minimal photobleaching and a much higher signal-to-noise ratio for real-time imaging in neurodegenerative settings. In addition to being an alternative to traditional immunocytochemistry, they provide the ability to visualize and track dynamic molecular processes over extended periods (e.g., from seconds to many minutes) (Tokuraku, Marquardt, and Ikezu 2009). The use of quantum dot labeling leads, for example to quantitatively measure the extent and thickness of glial scars, as in labeling and imaging of GFAP upregulation in gliosis, with a less diffuse labeling and higher nonspecific background (Silva 2009). Therefore, the use of this technology could also be particularly useful in the study of ALS (Choi, Lee, and Lee 2014).

3.2.4. Endogenous Fluorescent Animal Models in ALS

Progress in our understanding of neural organization and development has depended on a series of improvements in our ability to image individual neurons (Oglesby et al. 2012, Keller-Peck et al. 2001, Bridge et al. 2009). Endogenous fluorescent markers made it possible to monitor early pathological features and cell vulnerability in a variety of neurodegenerative diseases (Gatto et al. 2015). Still, some issues have to be considered while using endogenous fluorescent models of ALS, for example, the expression of different FPs has been documented as variable; therefore, it is important to compare conditions within the same founder line in which the expression remains stable.

In addition, a selective expression of fluorescent tags can be generated on different grey matter (GM) neurons making it possible to visualize a cell population or area. It should also be kept in mind that fluorescent brightness measured for a FP sample *in vitro* cannot be directly extrapolated to its actual brightness *in vivo*. Indeed, the resulting signal brightness generated by a FP expressed in living cells is determined not only by its intrinsic spectral characteristics, but also by parameters such as transcription and translation efficiency, mRNA and protein stability, and chromophore maturation rate (Chudakov et al. 2010).

In terms of fluorescently labeled upper motor neurons, the visualization and identification of neuron populations that show selective vulnerability, among thousands of different neuron populations within the heterogeneous and complex structure of the cerebral cortex, have been major limiting factors for success in bringing effective treatment strategies to neurodegenerative diseases such as ALS. Endogenous fluorescence has been used in invertebrate models to unveil the influence of different mutations and their influence on specific neuronal morphology (Sahin et al. 2017, Murakami et al. 2012). In murine models, the incorporation of fluorescent tags allow an unprecedented level of cellular detail in lower (Tallon et al. 2016) and upper motor neuron populations (Figure 2 & 3) (Genc and Ozdinler 2014, Genc et al. 2015). Specifically, the crossbreed of fluorescent mice with ALS transgenic mice is one of the microscopic pillars to assess, in more detail, complex cerebral structures (Figure 4). In that regard, the importance of analyzing cortical motor neurons has been emphasized by Genc et al. who generated a fluorescent mouse under the control of the ubiquitin C-terminal hydrolase-L1 (UCHL1) to visualize large pyramidal neurons located in layer V of the motor cortex. Using the proper animal breeding crosses with ALS animals, corticospinal motor neurons (CSMN) showed an initial vulnerability and a precise characterization of the timing and extension of the degenerative process (Genc and Ozdinler 2014). Using a similar fluorescent marker (GFP) in a SOD1 mouse at the peripheral region of the nervous system, Tallon et al. explored the "dying back" axonopathy (Tallon et al. 2016). Recently, additional cross-breed studies using yellow fluorescent protein (YFP) labels has been done to specifically evaluate the structural axonal changes in early stages of ALS (Gatto, Amin, et al. 2018). The finding from this double transgenic mouse (YFP, G93A- SOD1) has demonstrated the validity of this animal model to capture specific changes in white matter (WM) regions affected by the disease in detail.

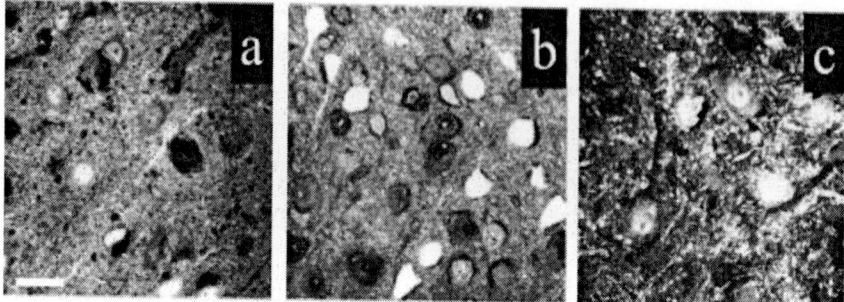

Figure 2. Evaluation of structural complexity across different grey matter of the central nervous system in a transgenic fluorescent mouse. a - Longitudinal section of the prefrontal cortex superficial (layers 1-3) grey matter (GM) region from a mouse expressing a yellow fluorescent protein (YFP). b - Evaluation of the hippocampus (deep GM region) Corpus Ammonis region one (CA1) from a YFP transgenic mouse. Pyramidal cells can be clearly observed in this animal model. c - Structural details from the spinal cord GM of the anterior horn labeled by YFP.

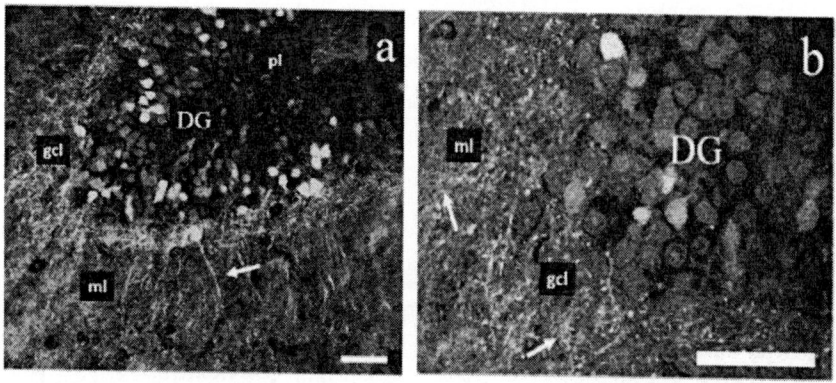

Figure 3. Ultrastructural imaging details of deep grey matter in a fluorescent transgenic mouse. a - Longitudinal section of the hippocampus dental gyrus (DG) demonstrating de degree of morphological detail in neuronal apical prolongations from the DG granular layer gcl (granular cell layer); pl (polymorphic layer, hilus) and ml (molecular layer) (arrow). Scale bar 10 microns. b - Higher magnification of a- showing larger fluorescent imaging details of the neuropil in the granular layer (arrows). Scale bar 10 microns.

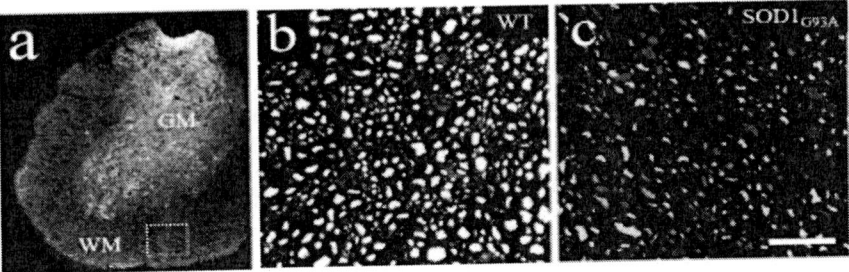

Figure 4. Assessment of central nervous system white matter structural anomalies in a murine fluorescent model of ALS. a - Cross-section of a lumbar spinal cord (SC) showing differences in grey matter (GM) and white matter (WM) in a transgenic ALS mouse model (SOD1$_{G93A}$) expressing a transgenic yellow fluorescence protein (YFP) tag. b - Higher magnification from a cross-section of the anterior WM region (doted square in a) showing axonal areas and extra-axonal space in the WT (b) or ALS mice (c).

3.3. Fluorescence Microscopy Methods

3.3.1. Confocal Microscopy in ALS

Conventional fluorescence microscopy is one of the most broadly used imaging techniques in cell biology. It enables straightforward observation of cellular structures and biomolecular dynamics with fluorophores or fluorescent proteins at the single-molecule level (Bolte and Cordelieres 2006).

In the biological sciences, the interaction of two molecular structures or proteins is often of key interest, and hence colocalization analysis is commonly performed. Colocalization refers to the geometric co-distribution of two fluorescent labels or color channels. Colocalization of two or more markers within these cellular structures may be defined as an overlap in the physical distribution of the molecular populations within a three-dimensional volume, this may be complete or partial; the main point is whether two fluorochromes are located on the same physical structure or on two distinct structures in a three-dimensional volume (Cordelieres and Bolte 2014). In many cases, the methods to analyze and score microscopic colocalization are often simple and descriptive rather than a quantitative assessment of the color overlay of two different fluorescent markers, with for instance green and red fluorescence resulting in a combination of two separate channel colors in case of colocalization (Adler and Parmryd 2010). Nevertheless, such a visual evaluation requires comparable fluorescence intensities of the two markers and is obviously far from being quantitative. Importantly, due to optical laws in image acquisition, in order to perform any colocalization analysis, this must be carried out in the three-dimensional space, and three-dimensional projections of image stacks must not be analyzed as they shrink volumetric information to two dimensions, leaving aside the depth component. These considerations led to calculating statistical parameters to evaluate the correlation of fluorescence-intensities of two (or more) detection channels on a pixel-by-pixel basis. Manders et al. proposed Pearson's correlation coefficient as a more quantitative measure of colocalization based on the pixel intensity correlation of two fluorescence channels (Moser et al. 2017). This is usually assessed over a whole region and metrically described using Pearson's correlation coefficient (PCC), Manders' overlap coefficient (MOC) and Manders' correlation coefficient (MCC) (Theart et al. 2018). All these calculations are very often performed in the Image J program using a tool named JACoP (Just Another Co-localization Plugin), that combines the currently used colocalization methods (Bolte and Cordelieres 2006). This technique has been widely used in confocal microscopy, and examples of these are the colocalization of proteins within aggregates. The level of colocalization is used qualitatively as well as quantitatively, as will be described in a later section.

Confocal microscopy images are also used in stereology analysis. Stereology is based on a set of statistical and mathematical principles and provides efficient tools for estimation of volume, surface area, length, and number of objects in 3-D structures by sampling in 2-D sections. It relies on statistical sampling principles and stochastic geometric theory aiming to prevent the limitations posed by assumptions about the 3-D structure of interest. Indeed, stereological estimations are the gold standard for quantitative studies of volume, length, and surface area as dimensional parameters in biomedical experiments (Kipanyula and Sife 2018).

In neuroscience, stereological methods are used more and more since qualitative scoring-based protocols are superficial and less reliable for use in studies of neuroprotection evaluations. The "Neurostereological" methods were developed to allow for unbiased total estimates of cell numbers in a specific brain region; these methods depend on the combination of estimators like the optical dissector and fractionator sampling scheme. This way, using an optimized neuro-stereology in conjunction with immunohistochemistry to label specific, biologically meaningful "markers" indicative of particular cell types, subclasses, or even states, allows for an assessment of the impact of neurological insults or disease progression on neuronal survival and neurodegeneration via quantification of absolute neuron and interneuron counts in various brain regions (Golub et al. 2015).

3.3.2. Latest Fluorescent Microscopy Techniques

Since current super-resolution microscopes are based on conventional optical imaging systems, improving the fundamental performance of the imaging systems can boost the spatial resolution and the image contrast of cell and sub-cellular structures (Dietz and Heilemann 2019, Lu, Vu, et al. 2019). Thus, aberration correction and adaptive optics, among others, are promising approaches to improve the imaging quality of optical systems (Fujita 2016). Super resolution microscopy (SRM) systems have been utilized in ALS animal research to determine the localization of protein aggregates (Schoen et al. 2015). However, in SRM the system is limited to 2D images because axially overlapped fluorophores cannot be separated. By introducing optical astigmatism, axial positions can be determined in a thin sample expanding the dimension to super-resolved 3D images (Lu, Tang, et al. 2019). The analysis of large 3D volumes is necessary for mapping the connections of far-reaching neurons inside the brain and determining the nature of cellular interactions underlying proper circuitry function and behavioral phenotype (Mano et al. 2018). This is performed with, light-sheet microscopy (LSM), which has proven to be a useful tool in neuroscience to image whole brains with high frame rates at cellular resolution; and, in combination with tissue clearing methods, the technique can be employed to reconstruct the cytoarchitecture over the intact optically cleared mouse brain (Mullenbroich et al. 2018) and might be an interesting tool to use in ALS research.

3.4. Microscopy Imaging Biomarkers in Preclinical Models of ALS

In this section we describe how different features of ALS are assayed (qualitatively or quantitatively) via the before mentioned microscopy techniques in the models previously described. The read out of these assays (imaging biomarkers) depict aggregation, neuroinflammation, innervation, motor neuron defects, neuronal loss and mis localization of proteins (Vijayakumar et al. 2019). We will describe them in an order that could be the sequence mechanism (though this not necessarily need be the case) leading to a final degeneration of motor neurons, denervation and muscular atrophy as schematically shown in (Figure 5).

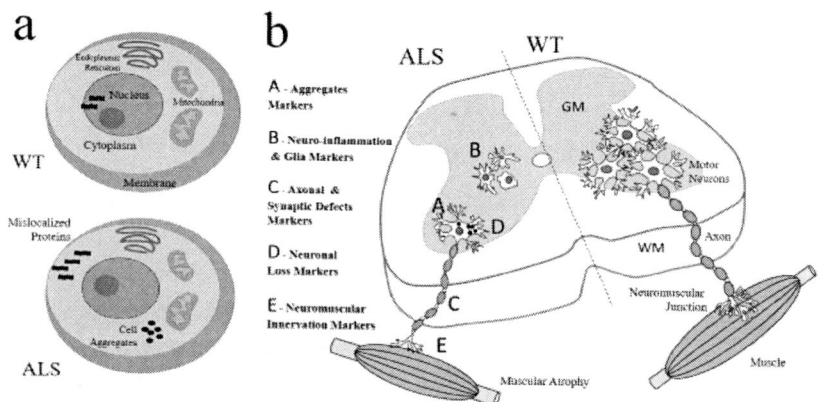

Figure 5. Scheme showing in vitro and ex vivo imaging biomarkers in ALS. a - Biomarkers that can be analyzed in single cells (*in vitro*), control (WT) and ALS models. b - Transversal section of a schematic spinal cord *(ex vivo)* showing structural biomarkers that can be analyzed in vertebrate models in control (WT, right) and their ALS counterparts (left). IMAGING BIOMARKERS: A - Aggregates: antibodies for proteins analyzed within an aggregate and possible colocalization with markers of post translational modifications (ubiquitin, phosphorylation); FISH for RNA foci. B - Neuroinflammation: Glia markers: astrocytes (GFAP, AQ4), microglia (CD68, Iba1), oligodendrocyte markers (MBP), lymphocyte (CD4+, CD8+) markers.
C - Motoneuron Defects: Stereology (cell number counting and volume determination) H&E, (Tubulin; NeuN,) apoptosis markers (TUNEL, caspase 3). D - Axonal connectivity: Neuron cytoskeleton markers (Neurofilament, MAP2).
E - Neuromuscular Innervation: Presynaptic (Synaptotagmin) & Postsynaptic (Ach receptors, alpha Bungarotoxin).

3.4.1. Aggregation, Inclusion and Foci Biomarkers

The presence of cytoplasmic inclusions or aggregates has been described in degenerating motor neurons and surrounding oligodendrocytes; not restricted to the spinal cord, but also present in other brain regions such as the frontal and temporal cortices, hippocampus, and cerebellum. The use of fluorescent dyes can be used for the detection of aggregates, inclusions or foci, which normally tends to be assessed in a qualitative manner (Oshinbolu et al. 2018).

Aggregation is a hallmark of pathology that is consistently recapitulated in yeast. It has proven especially useful in the analysis of FUS and TDP-43 proteinopathy, and yeast is an excellent platform for the discovery of protein-protein interactions (Di Gregorio and Duennwald 2018b). Shulin et al. used the yeast model to capture key aspects of molecular pathology. They used yeast strains expressing human FUS/TLS wild type and mutant forms N-terminally fused to green fluorescent protein (GFP) and showed FUS/TLS-associated proteotoxicity when the protein is mis-localized to the cytoplasm. They detected GFP signal in aggregates by fluorescence microscopy and showed, thus, that the model recapitulates the cytosolic aggregation and cytotoxicity observed in spinal motor neurons in the human disease (Ju et al. 2011). So did Sun et al. who associated FUS aggregates to toxicity in another YFP-tagged FUS yeast model (Sun et al. 2011). In addition, they analyzed the effects of truncations on FUS localization and defined C-terminal domains required for cytoplasmic localization and aggregation. They then showed that the domains of FUS required for aggregation in yeast contributed to aggregation in mammalian cells, using COS-7 and HEK cells, and an epifluorescent microscope with the criteria that only cells with greater than three foci under the YFP channel were considered as cells with aggregating FUS.

Regarding TDP-43 aggregates, Winton et al. demonstrated the presence of TDP-43 aggregates in HEK293 cells extracted to remove detergent-soluble pools of TDP-43. Their work demonstrated that a TDP-43 construct lacking the nuclear localization signal (NLS), mis-localized to the cytoplasm and also sequestered the endogenous TDP-43 to the cytoplasm in aggregates, not only in HEK cells, but also in hippocampal neurons, where neuronal accumulations, or aggregates of TDP-43 to similar to neuronal FTLD-U brains were observed (Winton et al. 2008).

Co-localization of FUS with aggregates on iPSC from patients with a FUS mutation showed that aberrant localization and recruitment of FUS into stress granules occurs only upon induction of stress in both, undifferentiated iPSCs and spinal cord neural cells (Lenzi et al. 2015). Using fluorescent antibodies against neurofilaments, Chen et al. quantified neurofilament inclusions in the cell bodies from cells of patients carrying a SOD1 mutation differentiated to motor neurons (Chen et al. 2014). And mutant TDP-43 iPSC-derived human neurons from an ALS patient revealed that the mutant cells had significantly higher levels of soluble and detergent-resistant TDP-43: cells expressing the mutant TDP-43 displayed predominantly nuclear TDP-43 localization with granular staining present in soma and neurites as shown by fluorescence microscopy (Bilican et al. 2012).

As far as studies in invertebrate models go, Baskoylu et al. determined the number and size of inclusions in *C. elegans* animals in a single-copy mutant SOD1 knock-in model. This is a non-overexpression model and thus helpful to gather information on a possible loss of function or gain of function mechanism. The work of Baskoylu et al. found that cholinergic and glutamatergic neurons are differentially sensitive to SOD-1 loss and gain of toxic function. In their work, human SOD1 inclusions were detected via their YFP fusion tag, and these were categorized according to size. *C. elegans* single-copy/knock-in models for mutants increased accumulation of the YFP-tagged human wild type SOD1 protein in small cytosolic inclusions, whereas *C. elegans* SOD1 inclusions were not increased in those with decreased SOD1 function, pointing to a gain of function mechanism. At the same time, SOD1 loss rendered glutamatergic neurons hypersensitive to oxidative stress (Baskoylu et al. 2018).

As an example of the analysis of the aggregation propensity of wild-type (WT) FUS in mice, Mitchell et al., overexpressed WT human FUS cDNA under the control of a mouse prion protein gene FUS+/+promoter. Mice developed a rapid decline in motor function from 4 weeks old, and displayed intense FUS perinuclear inclusions (Nolan, Talbot, and Ansorge 2016).

Aggregates were visualized by staining the hFUS protein and were visualized as ring-like inclusions (Mitchell et al. 2013).

Different proteins can be found in aggregates, and information on the composition of the aggregates described as colocalized to different markers in mouse models can be found in the study by Blokhuis (Blokhuis et al. 2013). Post translational modification of proteins in aggregates can also be assessed by colocalization of the marker that identifies the modification and a marker for aggregates such as ubiquitin present in aggregated ubiquitinated proteins (Richter-Landsberg 2007). Igaz et al. showed by double immunofluorescence, "extensive" colocalization of hyperphosphorylation markers and ubiquitin in TDP-43 aggregates in a transgenic mouse expressing human TDP-43 with a defective nuclear localization signal in the forebrain (Igaz et al. 2011).

Another type of aggregate, the Bunina bodies, the small, cystatin C-positive, eosinophilic cytoplasmic inclusions are generally considered a specific hallmark of sporadic ALS. These were also detected via staining against cystatin C in a TDP-43 transgenic primate non-human model by Uchida et al. (Uchida et al. 2012).

Inclusions containing RNA material, RNA inclusions, or foci point to RNA dysregulation and appears to be a major contributor to ALS pathogenesis. Indeed, TDP-43 and FUS are deeply involved in RNA processing such as transcription, alternative splicing and microRNA (miRNA) biogenesis (Butti and Patten 2018). (iPSC)-differentiated neurons from C9orf72 ALS patients, as an example, were analyzed via RNA FISH to exhibit clear intranuclear foci (Donnelly et al. 2013). Using FISH, Liu et al. also showed that sense and antisense RNA foci accumulate in mice from the C9-500 and C9-500/32 lines as early as 2 months of age, but not in C9-36/29, C9-37, or NT controls visualized in the brain and lumbar spinal cord sections via confocal microscopy (Liu et al. 2016).

3.4.2. Neuroinflammation Imaging Biomarkers

A hallmark of both familial and sporadic ALS is the presence of reactive immune cells in postmortem tissues, with microglial cells, the macrophages of the central nervous system (CNS), found in the vicinity of degenerating motor neuron cell bodies and axonal tracts (Chiot, Lobsiger, and Boillee 2019).

Many studies recognize that non-cell autonomous processes also contribute to motor neuron degeneration in certain rodent models and may also contribute to the sporadic form of ALS (Endo, Komine, and Yamanaka 2016). Investigated by different groups, markers for activated astrocytes (GFAP, ALDH1L1) and microglia (CD11b, CD68, Iba1) have been shown to increase throughout the stages analyzed in ALS mouse models (Philips and Robberecht 2011). As an example, Chiarotto et al. determined the expression of these markers in a G93A-SOD1 transgenic mouse model. By quantifying fixed regions of interest of the ventral horn of lumbar sections of spinal cords labeled with GFAP and Iba1 markers, they showed a decrease in astrogliosis and microglia activation after treatment with drugs tested at reducing neuroinflammation and ALS progression (Chiarotto et al. 2019). In addition, Aquaporin-4 (AQP4), the principal water channel protein in the mammalian central nervous system, localized on astrocyte processes and on ependymalcells might be used also as an interesting marker in ALS. This molecule provides a molecular pathway for water permeability and homeostasis in the brain and its astrocytic end-feet localization makes it a partner to blood-brain-barrier function, which has been documented more permeable in ALS. In that regard, studies by Nicaise et al. showed, in a SOD1 ALS transgenic rat model, overexpresion of this protein in astrocytes (Nicaise, Mitrecic, et al. 2009, Nicaise, Soyfoo, et al. 2009). The activation of these cells in ALS deep GM brain structures has been verified by immunohistochemical staining using an astrocytic marker on a YFP, G93A-SOD1 mouse by our research group (Figure 6).

In addition, other proteins involved in microglia activation that have received attention lately and that are being analyzed as possible ALS markers are chitinases, which have been measured in CSF (CHIT1, YKL-40), as well as macrophage chemo-attractant protein 1 (MCP-1) and shown to be elevated in ALS patients (Thompson and Turner 2019, Vu et al. 2020, Swash 2020). Another aspect that has gained attention is that of lymphocytes CD4+ and CD8+ infiltration. T cells in the CNS are rarely detected at early

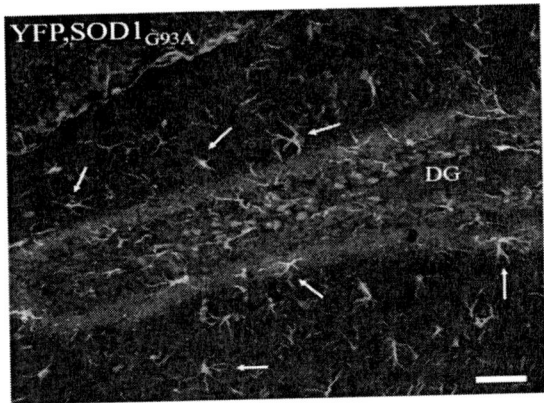

Figure 6. Glial imaging biomarkers assessed in a deep grey matter region from an ALS mouse. Immuno-histochemical staining (IHC) for the glia bioimaging marker acid fibrillary protein (GFAP) showing high astrocyte reactivity in the hippocampus dental gyrus (DG) of an ALS (SOD1$_{G93A}$) mouse. Scale bar = 10 microns.

disease stages, but readily infiltrate the spinal cord at later stages as disease progresses (Philips and Robberecht 2011, Liu and Wang 2017). However, their role has not been completely elucidated (Thompson and Turner 2019, Chiot, Lobsiger, and Boillee 2019). Oligodendrocytes have also been shown to be involved in the noncell-autonomous nature of ALS using mouse models of the disease (Ferraiuolo et al. 2011). Interestingly, through a motoneuron-oligodendrocyte coculture system, Ferraiuolo et al. showed oligodendrocytes derived from patients with familial and sporadic ALS from induced pluripotent stem cells and induced neural progenitor cells play an active role in MN death via soluble factors and cell-to-cell contacts. Markers for these cells being MBP and several enzymes involved in lipoproteins synthesis (Ferraiuolo et al. 2011). Alterations of these cells have also been described as "dysmorphic," with an increasing number of spinal cord oligodendrocytes showing a thickened, irregularly shaped cell body, enlarged cytoplasm and elongated reactive processes and in an apoptotic state (with caspase 3 expression, condensed chromatin, and dense clustering of reactive microglia around the degenerating oligodendrocyte); in addition, the myelin sheath composition is altered, with a prominent decrease in the levels of MBP, the second most abundant protein component of the myelin sheath, responsible for the formation, compaction and stabilization of myelin (Nonneman, Robberecht, and Van Den Bosch 2014).

3.4.3. Axonal and Synaptic Defects Biomarkers

Microscopy techniques are also instrumental in showing alterations within motor neurons providing markers for altered axonal transport, mislocalization of proteins, altered axonal branching or size, among others.

Due to the length of their axons, motor neurons are especially vulnerable to alterations that may affect the intracellular transport machinery. Axonal transport defects may thus be an important factor underlying the selective vulnerability of MNs or MN subtypes (Ragagnin et al. 2019). Altogether, intracellular trafficking defects, perturbations in motor proteins (Morfini et al. 2016), and the cytoskeleton (neurofilaments, peripherin, and posttranslational modification of these) contributes to aggregate formation, while aggregates disturb intracellular from and to ER-Golgi transport, nucleo-cytoplasmatic transport and axonal transport; but the precise molecular and functional details of these interactions remain to be dissected (Burk and Pasterkamp 2019). Thus, markers for the cytoskeleton, and molecular motors, which might be sequestered in aggregates or axonal "strangulation" are tools to analyze these events (Julien and Beaulieu 2000). Among these, neurofilaments and phosphorylated filaments have been a focus of attention as potential biomarkers in CSF for sporadic ALS (Verde, Silani, and Otto 2019, Poesen et al. 2017, Tsang et al. 2000).

In a zebra fish model carrying a TDP-43 ALS mutation, a staining with synaptic marker (synaptotagmin-1), was used to classify axonal defects via analysis of branching from microscope images (Lissouba et al. 2018). Nonspecific sterasas staining can be performed to assess muscle cells of varied sizes. Huang et al. used this method to determine changes in sizes in a TDP-43 transgenic rat model together with the ATP stain to show remodeling of motor neuron units leading to the conclusion in their work, that degenerating motor neurons cannot be rescued and that surviving motor units can be remodeled (Huang et al. 2012).

Axonal size can also be used to detect alterations by staining with neurofilament H. An increased numbers of small axons (<4 mm in diameter) was indicative of degeneration and regeneration, and fewer large caliber axons were counted via an Image J plugin in a C9orf72 expansion mutation mouse (Fischer et al. 2004). Lissouba et al. visualized abnormally shaped neurons via immunostaining against neurofilament (NF) and microtubule associated protein 2 (MAP2) as a dendritic marker on the cortex of Tbk1-NKO mice complemented with a Golgi-Cox staining to reveal a marked decrease in the density of dendritic spines and reduced dendritic spine density (Lissouba et al. 2018). In the transgenic TDP-43 monkey model, Uchida et al. showed the degeneration of motoneurons in areas where TDP-43 mis-localization to the cytoplasm had been detected. This was shown by loss of myelinated axons; the number and minimum diameters of neurons with nuclei in the lateral or medial nuclear groups in 15 sections evaluated after a Toluidine blue staining. In addition, the change in fiber type was assessed (Uchida et al. 2012).

As an example of axonal transport impairment or neuronal dying back pattern, wobble motor neurons were analyzed by electronmicrographs showing enlarged vesicles derived from the GARP (Pérez-Victoria et al. 2010). GARP dysfunction appears to have an impact on both the retrograde and the anterograde vesicle transport and might affect the integrity and function of the whole Golgi apparatus. Andrews et al. observed electron dense granular material in close proximity to the Golgi in degenerating wobbler motoneurons (Schmitt-John 2015).

Mis-localization of proteins is another important aspect to analyze in ALS models, and readily performed via microscopy using animal models aimed at recapitulating these features as present in patients. The experiments assaying this feature are those detecting the signal of the molecule of interest in the different cell compartments easily captured via microscopy. Many of the ALS-related mutant proteins are expressed in locations other than their normal one, especially TDP-43 and FUS. Uchida et al. was able to show, using a monkey model overexpressing the human TDP-43, the mis-localization of the TDP-43 protein (from nucleus to cytoplasm) in the lateral nuclear group of the spinal cord, that had not been recapitulated via any overexpressing TDP-43 transgenic rodent, fly, worm, or zebra fish models (Uchida et al. 2012). This localization and mis-localization, as well as hyperphosphorylation was detected via immunohistochemistry. Lenzi et al. quantified by immunostaining the intracellular localization of WT and mutant FUS proteins in iPSCs, thus obtaining the nuclear vs cytoplasmic signal level (Lenzi et al. 2015). The evaluation of the cortical neuronal morphology by confocal microscopy on the YFP, G93A-SOD1 mice has added an ultrastructural link between the molecular and ultrastructural neurodegenerative changes (Figure 7).

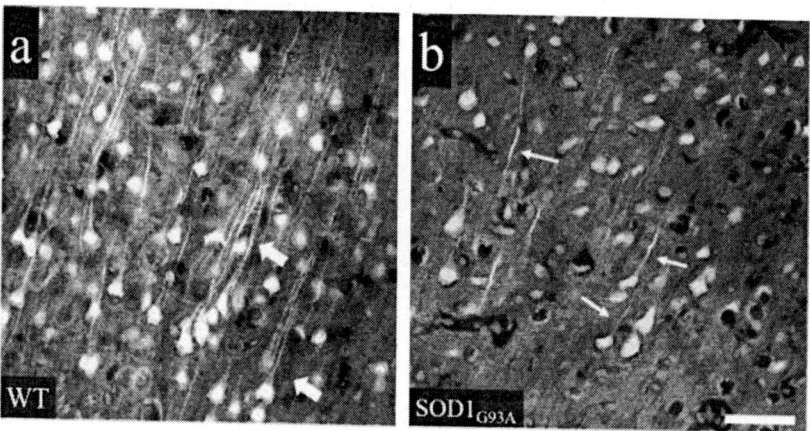

Figure 7. Cortical connectivity changes in an endogenous ALS fluorescent mouse model. Image of a longitudinal section from a prefrontal cortex in a mouse expressing YFP. Note the abundance of apical dendrites of pyramid cells (layer 3-5) in the control animal compared to the symptomatic ALS mice (arrows). Scale bar = 10 microns.

3.4.4. Neuronal Loss Biomarkers

In later stages of the disease, we find motoneuron death. This can be analyzed by staining and counting cells in control compared to ALS-models. The use of traditional staining methods remains a valuable tool in the analysis of cell loss. In transgenic mouse hTDP-43-NLS or hTDP-43-WT with the use of an H&E staining, numbers of neurons and, thus neuronal loss, was determined to show neuronal loss in selectively vulnerable forebrain regions, corticospinal tract degeneration, and motor spasticity recapitulating key aspects of FTLD and primary lateral sclerosis with the inducible transgene for the construct (Igaz et al. 2011). A significant loss in motor neurons counted as those stained by choline acetyltransferase (ChAT) or cresyl-violet staining of the lumbar spinal cord or Neu N staining was determined in a C9orf72 expansion mutation mouse (Fischer et al. 2004). Also, cell death occurring via apoptotic mechanism can be visualized via the TUNEL assay. In flies expressing glial hTDP-43, Krug et al. determined this by analyzing TUNEL positive cells (Krug et al. 2017).

In addition, the combination of cell staining with stereology yield robust data. As an example Mancuso et al. counted stained motoneurons with Cresyl Violet (Nissl Stain) to compare the number of motor neurons at different stages between two G93A-SOD1 strains in the lumbar spinal cord area (Mancuso et al. 2012). Using stereological principles to insure that every motor neuron in the lumbar spinal cord had an equal probability of being counted, neurons in the ventral horn with a distinct nucleolus and a darkly stained cytoplasm were manually traced using a volume criteria to count using an image software. This way, they determined motor neuron loss for the transgenic G93A-SOD1 mouse compared to the control at the time points analyzed (Fischer et al. 2004). Tong et al. used a transgenic rat model that expresses a mutant form of human TDP-43 restricted to astrocytes to show -via stereological methods- that the selective expression of mutant TDP-43 in astrocytes caused a progressive loss of motor neurons and the denervation atrophy of skeletal muscles, resulting in progressive paralysis (Tong et al. 2013). Uchida et al. through their stereological analysis of cell counts in non-human primate model, detected neuronal loss associated to TDP-43 mis-localization in almost all the large motoneurons of the lateral nuclear group at the early or even the presymptomatic stage. Incidentally, this mis-localization could only be detected in this model and not reproduced in any rodent model (Uchida et al. 2012).

Cell loss can, but not necessarily, lead to volume reduction. Linares et al. examined the volumes of lumbar spinal cord sections from transgenic mutant SOD1 rat models stained with Toluidine blue and acetyl choline transferase (ChaT) markers to quantify cell numbers and section volumes (Linares et al. 2013). Lu et al. quantified the number of NeuN positive cells in different segments of spinal cord sections to analyze the neuronal loss in a G93A-SOD1 mouse model at different stages and TDP-43 positive cells (in neurons and oligodendrocytes), to determine that the amount of TDP-43 positive cell is cervical>lumbar>thoracic, and that its increase correlates with an increase in neuronal death (Lu et al. 2016). Huang et al. used this method to determine average size of motor neurons in L3–L5 cords and the total volume of the ventral horns of L3–L5 cord in an overexpressing TDP-43 rat model. They detected more than 60% of spinal motor neurons loss in mutant TDP-43 transgenic rats at disease end stages with unaltered volume of ventral lumbar cords (Huang et al. 2012).

3.4.5. Imaging Biomarkers of Neuromuscular Innervation

The events previously described lead to neuromuscular junction (NMJ) disruption (Dadon-Nachum, Melamed, and Offen 2011, Dupuis and Loeffler 2009, Tremblay, Martineau, and Robitaille 2017, Wymer and Borchelt 2018). Tallon et al. quantified the percentage of NMJ innervation in a WT and SOD1 fluorescent mouse model via the overlap of presynaptic and postsynaptic markers, using the YFP signal (expressed in all motor neurons) to identify the NMJ, and bungarotoxin antibody as a postsynaptic marker (AChRs) in the lateral thoracic nerve (LTN) and the cutaneous maximus muscle (CMM) system (Tallon et al. 2016). The analysis was performed on confocal z-stack flattened images.

Denervation was also detected by Brenner et al. in immunofluorescent muscle and spinal cord sections, using a confocal microscope, and determining the overlap of the pre-synapse (neurofilaments, synaptophysin) and the post-synapse (a-bungarotoxin; fully innervated, partially innervated, fully denervated) using the ImageJ "Maximum projection" function. NMJs were assessed as "denervated" when presynaptic synaptophysin/ neurofilament staining was completely absent in the G93A-SOD1 Tbk1+/- mice and controls (Brenner et al. 2019) (Liu et al. 2016). Also, using scores, Fischer et al. obtained "innervated" as a complete overlap with the axon terminal, or "denervated" if the endplate was not associated with an axon. If the neuromuscular junctions were associated with a preterminal axon only or showed partial overlap between end-plate and terminal, were labeled "intermediate" (Fischer et al. 2004). Liu et al. also quantified denervation in the neuromuscular junctions in the tibialis anterior and diaphragm muscles of a C9orf72 expansion mutation mouse to determine a higher number of the transgenic versus the non-transgenic animal (using a marker for acetylcholine receptors (bungarotoxin labeled) and synapse (neurofilament H) (Fischer et al. 2004).

4. MRI Diffussion in ALS

In addition to the critical advances in optical imaging techniques, magnetic resonance imaging (MRI) has been increasingly available in the study of preclinical models in neurosciences due to the high spatial resolution and the advantage of the technique being non-invasive. Magnetic resonance provides a unique opportunity to quantify the diffusional characteristics of a wide range of specimens. Because diffusional processes are influenced by the geometrical structure of the environment, MRI can be used to probe the structural environment non-invasively (Johansen-Berg and Behrens 2014). From the conventional volumetric methods using T2-weighted MRI images, a significant amount of progress has been done during the last decades to refine and define useful marker of ALS pathology to monitor disease evolution (Comi, Rovaris, and Leocani 1999). Recently, the use of high and ultra-high magnetic fields has significantly increased resolution as well as sensitivity and specificity in the detection of microstructural anomalies across different preclinical models of ALS (Gatto, Amin, et al. 2019, Gatto, Amin, et al. 2018). Ultimately, the multimodal combination of imaging technologies and advancement in computational methods such as artificial intelligence and machine learning algorithms are accelerating and helping to understand the microstructural changes as well as improving the detection possibilities of the disease at earlier stages (Querin et al. 2018, Borsodi et al. 2017).

4.1. Fundamentals in MRI Diffusion

Magnetic resonance is based upon the interaction between an applied magnetic field and a particle that possesses spin and charge. The magnetic field can be represented as a vector, meaning that it has both a magnitude and a direction that is proportional to the current applied to the system. Specifically, a short burst of radiofrequency (RF) energy (typically a narrow range or bandwidth centered around a central frequency) is applied to the samples. During the pulse, the protons absorb a portion of this energy which influences another property of the nucleus called spin or intrinsic spin angular momentum. When the RF transmitter is turned off, the protons immediately begin to realign and return to their original equilibrium orientation emitting their energy at a specific peak amplitude, frequency and phase related to the strength of the initially applied magnetic field. Further mathematical processing can map the signals and obtain the object image (Dale et al. 2015). Among all the atoms found in biology, the hydrogen nucleus, consisting of a single proton, is a natural choice for probing the body using MRI technique due to its abundance in tissue components such as water and fat.

MRI provides a unique opportunity to quantify the diffusional characteristics of a wide range of specimens because diffusional processes are influenced by the geometrical structure of the environment, and MRI can be used to probe the structural environment non-invasively (Gatto, Chauhan, and Chauhan 2015, Gatto and Weissmann 2019, Gao et al. 2020). Considering a probabilistic model to describe the motion of an ensemble of particles undergoing diffusion, we could quantify the fraction of particles that will traverse a certain distance within a particular timeframe, mathematically speaking, the likelihood that a single given particle will undergo that displacement. For example, in free diffusion, the displacement distribution is theoretically represented by a Gaussian function whose width is determined by the diffusion coefficient. However, in inhomogeneous and porous media, such as that found in biological tissues, non-Gaussian models could provide a more representative function of the real tissue complexity, as explained in the following sections.

Using fast and efficient pulse sequences, diffusion MRI (dMRI) can quickly identify defects or damage to soft tissue with high resolution and contrast. dMRI is complementary to T1 and T2 relaxation contrast due to its sensitivity to the translational diffusion of water at the micron length scale of cells. Hence, dMRI, can identify tissue changes in intracellular, extracellular, and vascular compartments via the selective reduction in signal intensity at high, intermediate, and low b-values (strength of the gradient magnetic field) (Magin et al. 2019).

4.2. Uncompartmentalized Models (Diffusion Tensor Imaging)

Considered in its simplest terms, diffusion-weighted MRI measures the net displacement of water molecules in a voxel over a few milliseconds. By measuring the degree and direction of diffusion, the structure of the local environment across diffusing molecules can be determined (Lipton 2008). Thus, if the molecules interact with a boundary, such as cell membranes, the MRI signal will be altered. Overall, such boundaries will give rise to both hindered and restricted diffusion, which is often attributed to water trapped within and between cells, respectively. In brain tissue, for example, diffusing molecules will travel several microns during a diffusion measurement. This means that the diffusion signal is most sensitive to changes in microstructure within this spatial scale range (Van Hecke et al. 2016, Kingsley 2006).

Diffusion tensor imaging (DTI) expands these concepts further by modeling diffusion as a mathematical tensor, describing the amount and direction of diffusion in each voxel related to the gradient direction. Specifically, DTI is based on the diffusion tensor reconstruction, which is obtained by combining diffusion measurements along at least six non-collinear spatial directions and it can be described as a mono-exponential decay using the Stejskal-Tanner equation (Le Bihan et al. 2001, Kingsley 2006), which has been fundamental to distinguish differences between control and ALS animals (Figure 8). This is performed to characterize the orientation-dependent water mobility in each voxel, and to correlate it with the tissue architecture, parametric maps in *ex vivo* perfused samples (Figure 9) and more importantly, during *in vivo* experiments (Figure 10). DTI indices provide information about the underlying microstructural characteristics of biological tissues (Soares et al. 2013). In general terms, the methods to analyze DTI can be divided into the following categories: region of interest (ROI),(Froeling, Pullens, and Leemans 2016) voxel-based analysis (VBA),(Abe et al. 2010, Chen et al. 2018) tract-based spatial statistics (TBSS),(Smith et al. 2006) and fiber tractography)(Agosta et al. 2010, Fujiyoshi et al. 2013, Calabrese et al. 2015, Basser et al. 2000) (See Figure 9). A popular used metric in research studies is fractional anisotropy (FA), which characterizes the degree of anisotropy in each voxel describing the general status of the underlying tissue architecture (Tournier, Mori, and Leemans 2011). The use of DTI to study microstructural changes in transgenic animal models of ALS has been growing significantly. Overall, rodent models are the most used due to comparative fastest life cycle and low cost and most of the preclinical studies rely on high and ultra-high field MRI increasing imaging resolution (Table 2) (Cardenas et al. 2017, Gatto, Amin, et al. 2018, Gatto, Amin, et al. 2019).

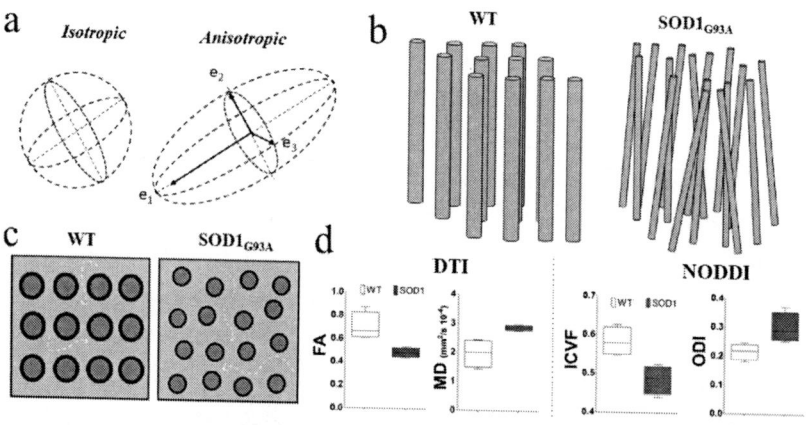

Figure 8. Diagram showing different aspects of mono and multi-compartmental models of structural diffusion MRI. a - Diagram of two MRI diffusion patterns. The extracted *eigenvalues* can account for the microstructural changes in the biological tissues of the central nervous system derived from to the ALS pathology. b - Three-dimensional representation of axonal tracts in white matter (WM) tissues. c - Transversal section scheme of tracts from b showing the WM compartmental redistribution during the progression of ALS. d - Parameters obtained from diffusion tensor imaging (DTI) such as fractional anisotropy (FA) and mean diffusion (MD) can be applied to measure axonal integrity (mono-compartmental model). Multicompartmental models, such as neurite orientation dispersion and density imaging (NODDI) can estimate WM changes in the intracellular compartment through the intracellular volume fraction component (ICVF) and extracellular partition thorugh the orientation density index (ODI). Example of DTI and NODDI outputs from the corpus callosum genu in control and ALS are presented.

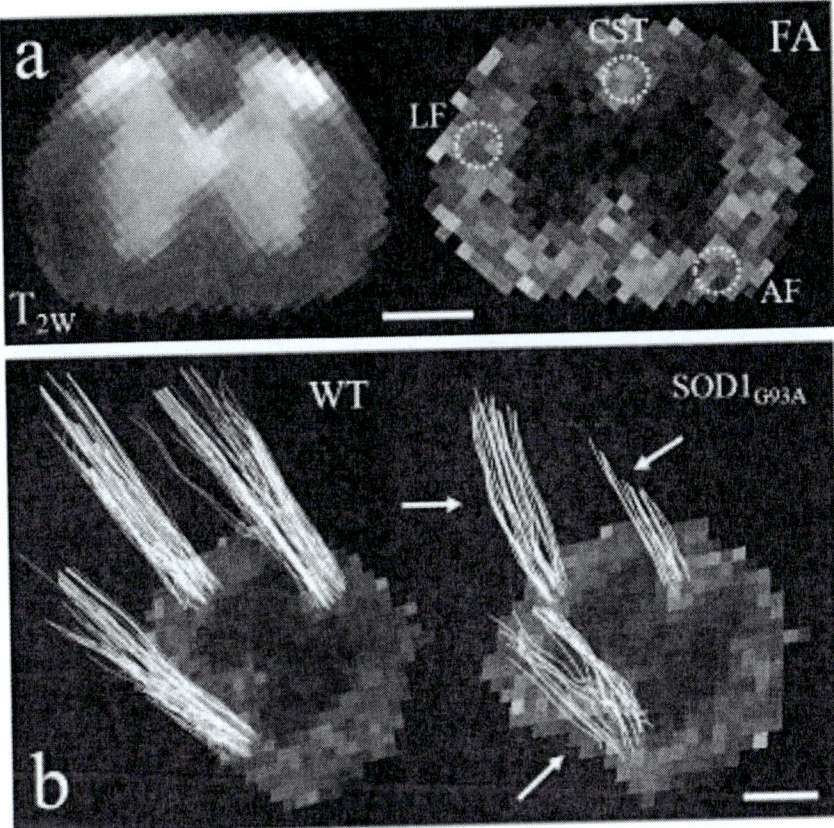

Figure 9. Ex vivo spinal cord microstructural and tractography white matter changes in a murine model of ALS at 16.7T. a - Anatomical (T2w) and fractional anisotropy (FA) map from a mouse lumbar spinal cord *(ex vivo)* section are presented. Three regions of interest are segmented across different white matter regions (dotted circular areas). b - Probabilistic tractography calculation across different funiculi (WM segments from a) showing significant differences in fiber reconstruction between WT (control) and ALS mice (SOD1-G93A). Note the different susceptibility between WM tract locations in the ALS mice (arrows). Scale bar = 1 millimeter.
Abbreviations: CST, Cortical Spinal Tract; LF, Lateral Funiculi; AF, Anterior Funiculi; SC, Spinal cord.

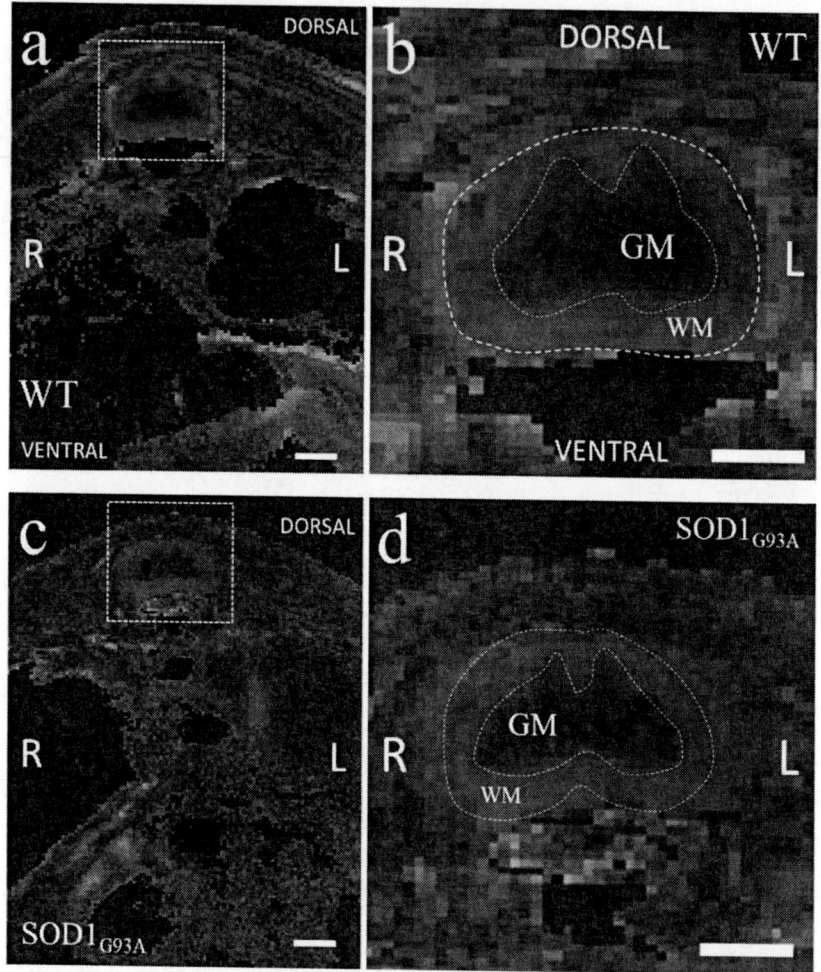

Figure 10. In vivo assessment of a lumbar section of the spinal cord from a control and ALS mouse at 9.4T. a - Diffusion tensor imaging (DTI) and a fractional anisotropy (FA) map showing a transversal abdominal section at the level of the lumbar spinal cord (dotted squares) in a control mouse. Scale bar = 2 millimeter. b - Zoomed image from a showing macrostructural details of the spinal cord white (WM) and grey matter (GM) (marked in doted line) as well as the microstructure (FA map). c - Comparative illustration from a symptomatic ALS mouse. d – Magnified SC area showing a reduction in WM and GM volumes. Scale bar = 2 millimeter.
Abbreviations: R, right; L, left; WT, GM, grey matter, WM, white matter; WT, wild type; SOD1-G93A, ALS mice.

Table 2. Summary of DTI studies in murine models of ALS

Study	Animal model	Age	Field Strength	CNS Structures	Parameters	Results (ALS vs. Control)
Gatto et al. 2019 (ex vivo)	C57-G93A-SOD1 vs WT (n=4 per group)	P60, P80, P120	17.6T	CC, Hipp and CCX (FrAx, Cing, M1, M2, S1, S2, Au, Vis)	FA, AD, RD, ADC	CC, CCX - Decreased FA CC - Increased in RD and CCX MD Hipp - Decreased FA, Increased RD and MD
Muller et al. 2019 (in vivo)	TDP-43 vs WT (n=10 per group)	20 wks	11.7T	Brain M1/M2 CST, CC	FA, AD, RD, MD	Decreased FA NS change in AD Increased RD & MD
Gatto et al. 2018c (ex vivo)	C57-G93A-SOD1 vs WT (n=5 per group)	P80 and P120	17.6T	SCwm (L, Tx, C)	FA, AD, RD, ADC	SCwm - Decreased in FA, AD SCwm - Decrease in RD, ADC
Gatto et al. 2018b (in vivo)	C57-G93A-SOD1 vs WT (n=5 per group)	P80 and P120	9.4T	SCwm	ADC, FA, AD	SCwm - Decreased FA, AD SCwm - Increased ADC, RD
Gatto et al. 2018a (ex vivo)	B6Jl-G93A-SOD1 vs WT (n=5 per group)	P80 and P120	9.4T	SCwm, and SCgm	FA, AD, RD, MD	SCwm - Decreased FA, AD SCwm - Increased RD, MD SCgm - Increased FA SCgm - Decreased AD, RD, MD
Mancuzzo et al. 2017 (in vivo)	G93A-SOD1 vs WT (n=5 per group)	7,8,10,12,15 wks	7T	SCwm, and SCgm	AD, RD, MD	SCwm - Decreased FA, AD and MD SCwm - NS chance in RD SCgm - Decreased AD and MD
Figini et al. 2016 (in vivo)	G93A-SOD1 vs WT (n=5 per group)	10,17 wks	7T	SCwm, and SCgm	FA, AD, RD, MD	SCwn and SCgm Decreased FA, AD, MD Variable change in RD SCgm - Decreased RD

Table 2. Summary of DTI studies in murine models of ALS (cont.)

Study	Animal model	Age	Field Strength	CNS Structures	Parameters	Results (ALS vs. Control)
Caron et al. 2015 (ex vivo)	C57-G93A-SOD1[1] 129Sv-G93A-SOD1[2] vs WT (n=4 per group)	15,19,22 wks[1] 14,15,16 wks[2]	7T	SC ventrolateral MNs	FA and AD	SC – Decreased FA and AD
Kim et al. 2013 (in vivo)	G93A-SOD1 vs WT (n=5 per group)	10 wks	4.7T	SC ventrolateral MNs & BN (VII and XII)	ADC, FA, AD, RD	BN - Decreased ADC, FA & Increased AD SC – Decreased ADC, FA and AD & Increased RD
Underwood et al. 2010 (in vivo)	G93A-SOD1 vs WT (n = 6 per group)	P45, P75, P110, P145	16.4T	SC ventrolateral WM	FA, AD, RD	Decreased FA and AD Increased RD
Kim et al. 2010 (in vivo)	G93A-SOD1 vs WT (n=5 per group)	12 wks	4.7T	SC ventrolateral MNs &BN (VII and XII)	ADC, FA, AD, RD	BN - Decreased in ADC SC- Decreased in FA and AD SC - Increased in RD SC - NS in ADC
Niessen et al. 2006 (in vivo)	B6Jl-G93A-SOD1 vs WT (n=4 vs n=5)	P70 & P90	4.7T	SC, CCX & Th, BN V, VII XII	ADC	CCX, BN V, VII, XII - Increased ADC SC - NS in ADC

Abbreviations: CCX. cortex; CC, Corpus Callosum; Hipp., hippocampus. SC, Spinal Cord; SCwm, Spinal Cord white matter; SCgm, Spinal Cord grey matter; BN, brainstem nucleus;Th, Thalamus; CST, Cortico-Spinal tract; M1 cortical motor area 1; M2 cortical supplementary motor area 2; L, Lumbar Segment; Tx, Thoracic Segment; C, Cervical segment; MNS, motoneurons; ADC, Apparent Diffusion Coefficient; FA, Fractional Anisotropy; AD, Axial Diffusion; RD, Radial Diffusion; MD, Mean Diffusion; WT, wild type; P, postnatal day; wks, weeks; ND, non-significant; T, Tesla magnetic field.

4.3. Multicompartmental Diffusion Models

To estimate parameters with even more neurobiological relevance, we need biophysical models that account for the changes in diffusion parameters as a consequence of the combination of diffusion signals from distinguishable water compartments: a signal representing the intra-cellular compartment and an additional one the extra-cellular compartment. Despite its importance in brain function, the morphology of the extracellular space (ECS) on the submicron scale is largely unknown. However, using MRI diffusion techniques with additional gradient diffusion values it is possible to extract the extracellular volume fraction, which captures the fraction of total tissue volume that lies outside of cells (Johansen-Berg and Behrens 2014). Among diverse multicompartment models proposed, we can mention AxCaliber (AxCal) (Assaf et al. 2008, Barazany, Basser, and Assaf 2009), Diffusion Basis Spectrum Imaging (DBSI) (Wang et al. 2014) and Restriction Spectrum Imaging (RSI) (Reas et al. 2017, Sowa et al. 2019), the Neurite orientation dispersion and density imaging (NODDI); the latter has gained popularity due to its easy and robust implementation methods (Zhang et al. 2012).

In NODDI, the diffusion signal is decomposed into three different compartments: 1) a restricted compartment anisotropic Gaussian diffusion with zero radial diffusivity (referred to as the intra-neurite space); 2) a hindered compartment of anisotropic Gaussian diffusion with nonzero radial diffusivity related to neurite density via the tortuosity model (referred to as the extra-neurite space) and 3) free water (isotropic Gaussian diffusion) paralleling cerebrospinal fluid (CSF) (Wang et al. 2019, Zhang et al. 2012). NODDI, extensively used in medicine (Broad et al. 2019, Zhang et al. 2018, Kamagata, Hatano, and Aoki 2016) and neuroscience (Sato et al. 2017, McCunn et al. 2019), has proved to have a higher sensitivity and greater tissue specificity to identify WM abnormalities across different compartments compared with conventional DTI in presymptomatic ALS patients (Wen et al. 2019). Moreover, parameters such as neurite dispersion index (NDI) and Orientation Dispersion Index (ODI) have been detected showing changes in deep GM structures (bulbar GM) as well as disease duration (Broad et al. 2019). This compartmental redistribution captured by NODDI has been recently validated by histological analyses in SOD1 mouse models (Gatto, Mustafi, et al. 2018), facilitating the analysis of neurite morphology and quantification of the altered CNS structures during very early stages of the disease (Gatto, Amin, et al. 2019).

4.4. Anomalous Diffusion Models

The mobility of water in biological tissues is not completely random, but is hindered and restricted by cellular and sub-cellular tissue structure, as well as by the extracellular matrix of proteoglycans and fibrous proteins (Gatto, Li, et al. 2018). This requires mathematical models with parameters reflecting features of the cellular organization of the tissue and its composition (Magin et al. 2019). Considering the heterogeneous nature of biological tissues in health and disease it is logical to think that diffusion is not always Gaussian (Hofling and Franosch 2013). Hence, several approaches have been suggested to provide a deeper insight into the diffusion phenomenon. As an example, the measurements of tortuosity and tissue organization through the ECS are distributed to geometric inhomogeneities and interactions in a semi restrictive diffusion regime (so-called hindered compartment). One of the most popular non-Gaussian models is the diffusional kurtosis imaging (DKI) model (Jensen et al. 2005, Arab et al. 2018). In this model, the deviation from Gaussian behavior is quantified using convenient dimensionless metrics (Jensen and Helpern 2010). Recent research in SOD1 mice using this imaging technique demonstrated broader and earlier WM and GM reductions in the mean kurtosis (MK) metric, possibly related to the decrease in neuronal complexity (Gatto, Amin, et al. 2019). Further clinical studies have shown a similar reduction in DKI parameters and indicates similar decreases in the microstructural complexity in ALS patients as observed in the preclinical models (Figure 11) (Welton et al. 2019, Huang et al. 2020).

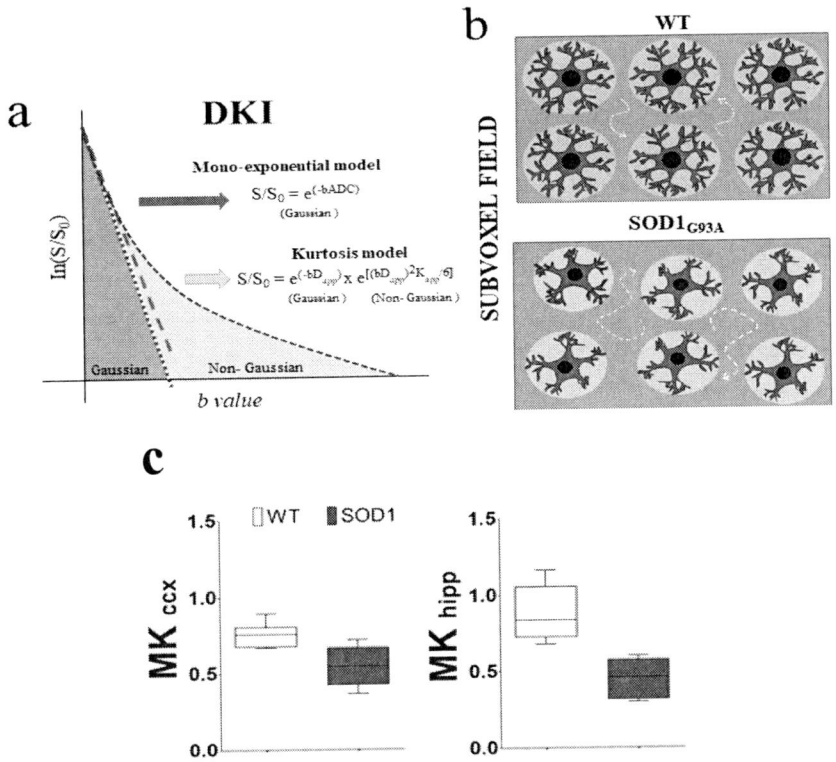

Figure 11. Scheme demonstrating different aspects of MRI anomalous diffusion models in the context of ALS. a - Diagram of the differences between MRI Gaussian and non-Gaussian diffusion models (Kurtosis diffusion model). b - Scheme representing two different diffusion environments: extracellular-non restricted Gaussian diffusion regime and a more restricted (hindered) non-Gaussian diffusion environment. Note that, as the grey matter (GM) decreases in complexity due to the progression of the disease, a change can be detected between these compartments. c - Mean kurtosis (MK) sample plots (non-Gaussian Model) from superficial GM and deep GM comparing the decrease of complexity between WT (control) and ALS mice (SOD1). Abbreviations: MKCCX, mean Kurtosis from prefrontal cortical area; MKhipp, mean Kurtosis from hippocampus (deep GM).

Additional non-Gaussian models can interrogate the complex biological tissues (membranes, organelles, and cells). In a very simplistic approach, several recent studies have investigated the so-called anomalous diffusion stretched exponential model where α is a measure of tissue complexity that can be derived from fractal models of tissue structure (Bennett et al. 2003, Ito, Ogura, and Tomisaki 1992). Increasing complexity, diffusion can be interpreted based on perturbations in the motion of the water molecules in proton MRI that entwines structure with statistics. Specifically, diffusivity calculations in this model are done via power law generalizations of the classical Brownian pattern, introducing halts between steps (waiting times) and restrictions on step sizes (jump lengths). This generalization is formally incorporated into the analysis of MRI diffusion data as the Continuous Time Random Walk (CTRW) model (Magin et al. 2013). From this approach fractional order parameters α and β, have been used to describe tissue complexity, heterogeneity, and tortuosity providing new biomarkers that encode tissue complexity as observed in other models of neurodegenerative diseases and potentially useful in the interrogation of ALS (Gatto, Ye, et al. 2019).

Recently, fractal order calculus model (FROC) has been developed for the characterization of anomalous diffusion in MRI resulting in a simpler, computationally faster, and more direct way to incorporate tissue complexity and microstructure into diffusional dynamics (Liang et al. 2016). However, drawbacks to the use of such anomalous diffusion models are the need for high b values and lengthy acquisition time, as well as computational complexity. New techniques such as quasi-diffusion imaging (QDI), are able to compress the acquisition of multi-shell b-value diffusion data using shorter acquisition times, (Barrick et al. 2020), but its potential to capture complexity in preclinical ALS tissue is still to be determined (De Giorgio et al. 2019, Gois et al. 2020).

4.5. Correlative Multi-Imaging Biomarkers Assessment

The development of new approaches to slow down the evolution in ALS requires the identification of robust biomarkers for disease activity that provide an earlier diagnosis and perhaps lead to improved prognosis (Turner et al. 2011). While optical and fluorescence microscopy offers a superior imaging resolution, MRI imaging can acquire signals from physiologically intact organisms. Therefore, the combination of optical and MRI techniques offers the best of both worlds with a comprehensive and scalable assessment of molecular, microstructural, and volumetric imaging variables (Table 3). In the SOD1 mice spinal cord, the evaluation of MRI diffusion parameters can be sub-divided towards specific structures from different cellular populations. Key genetic mutations in ALS induce changes in tissue structure and organization of intercellular scaffold proteins like collagen or other active proteins related to transmembrane water transport (aquaporins), among others. Recently, our *in vivo* MRI studies have been able to demonstrate that apparent diffusion coefficients (ADC) are temporarily related to microstructural anomalies on some bioimaging markers described earlier, particularly at very early stages of the disease (Gatto, Li, et al. 2018, Niessen et al. 2006). Diffusion techniques, such as DTI, Fractional Anisotropy (FA) and axial diffusion (AD) can yield information related to structural markers of axonal integrity (Alba-Ferrara and de Erausquin 2013), such as intracellular neurofilament staining markers (SMI-31) (Gatto, Li, and Magin 2018) or YFP labeled axons (Gatto 2018). The role of membrane insulation by oligodendrocytes, present in WM, has been studied in different animal models of demyelination (Field et al. 2019, Torre-Fuentes et al. 2020), as well as in the context of ALS (Kang et al. 2013, Ludolph 2013, Nonneman, Robberecht, and Van Den Bosch 2014). Similarly, G93A-SOD1 mice exhibit similar myelin alterations at early stages of the disease detected by a decrease in radial diffusivity (RD) indicating its additional role in ALS and the possibility to use this parameter as a valuable predictive marker of disease progression. As an example, some of this DTI markers have been used to follow therapeutic efficacy of stem cell transplantation in the SOD1 mice (Bontempi et al. 2018). As previously mentioned, one additional advantage of MRI diffusion is the possibility to use a tensor approach to generate a mathematical probabilistic reconstruction of WM fibers (Sarica et al. 2014, Mori et al. 1999, Basser et al. 2000). Efforts to validate this technique have been attempted using neuronal tracers (Calabrese et al. 2015, Aydogan et al. 2018), still several geometrical inaccuracies have not been fully resolved (Mukherjee et al. 2008, Daducci et al. 2016). Thus, future research directions might focus in improving the MRI resolution capacity

Table 3. Microstructural MRI diffusion parameters and optical microscopy imaging biomarkers in murine models of ALS

MRI Bioimaging Marker (WM)		Biological Attribute	Presymptomatic	Symptomatic	Molecular & Structural Biomarker
DTI	ADC	Tissue scaffold structure	Unchanged	Increased ↑↑	Collagen (Ono et al. 1998, Gatto, Li, et al. 2018) AQP4 (Bataveljic et al. 2012, Gatto, Amin, et al. 2018)
	RD	Oligodendrocytes - Myelin Content	Increased ↑↑	Decrease ↑↑↑	MBP (Gatto, Li, and Magin 2018, Gatto, Mustafi, et al. 2018)
	AD	Axonal Degeneration	Decrease ↓↓	Unchanged	YFP (Axons) (Gatto, Li, et al. 2018)
	FA	Axonal Integrity	Decreased ↓	Decreased ↓↓	SMI-31(Gatto 2018, Gatto, Li, and Magin 2018) SMI-32 (Kim et al. 2011) (WM) NeuN & ChAT (Gatto, Li, and Magin 2018) (GM) YFP (Axons) (Gatto 2018, Gatto, Li, et al. 2018)
NODDI	ICVF	Intracellular compartment	Decreased ↓	Decreased ↓↓	YFP (Axons) (Gatto et al. 2018)
	ODI	Extracellular compartment	Increased ↑	Increased ↑↑	YFP (Extra-axonal Space) (Gatto, Mustafi, et al. 2018)
DKI	MK (GM)	Neuronal complexity	Decreased ↓	Decreased ↓↓	YFP (Neuronal Bodies) (Gatto, Amin, et al. 2019, Gatto 2020)

Abbreviations: WM, White Matter; GM, Grey Matter; DTI, diffusion tensor Imaging; NODDI, Neurite Orientation Dispersion and Density Imaging; ICVF, Intracellular Volume fraction; ODI, Orientation Dispersion index; DKI, Diffusion Kurtosis Imaging; ADC, Apparent Diffusion Coefficient; FA, Fractional Anisotropy; AD, Axial Diffusion; RD, Radial Diffusion; MD, Mean Diffusion; MK, Mean Kurrtosis; YFP, Yellow Fluorescent Protein, MBP Myelin Basic Protein; AQP-4, Aquaporin-4; ChAT, Choline Acetyltransferase; SMI-31, phosphorylated neurofilament H; SMI-32, nonphosphorylated neurofilament H; NeuN, Fox-3, Rbfox3, or Hexaribonucleotide Binding Protein-3

and use a more methodical approach to constantly validate diffusion variables with a proper bioimaging marker. Ultimately, all the different mathematical models presented have inherent pitfalls when they are compared to any histological template (Thomas et al. 2014, Vedantam et al. 2013). Thus, a more holistic approach, (Gatto, Amin, et al. 2019) resulting from the combination of different diffusion models together with histological assays might be better suited to unveil the right research model and yield a better link between the preclinical and clinical ALS fields.

CONCLUSION

During the last decades, experimental animal models have improved our understanding of different pathogenic mechanisms involved in ALS. In addition, new advances in neuroimaging have led to higher imaging resolution outputs and the possibility to test potential therapeutic strategies. The different imaging modalities (optical and MRI tecniques) analysed have advantages and disadvantages based on the intrinsic physical signal resolution and ability to capture physiological changes in intact organisms. Recently new transgenic endogenous fluorescent animal models have provided a means to assess the ultrastructural changes related to genetic mutations and improve our understanding of the links between molecular mechanism and brain tissue microstructures. A possible *in vivo* approach that we envision is the use of multi-modal imaging methods, combining the analysis of optical fluorescent methods with specific and novel MRI diffusion models. This way, the improved technologies acquired in the ALS field may lead to a better understanding of the pathophysiology of the disease and therefore to the design of effective therapeutics.

ACKNOWLEDGMENTS

We would like to thank Dr. Richard Magin for his suggestions and proofreading of the MRI section of this mansucurpt and Dr. Osvaldo Uchitel for his feedback.

REFERENCES

Abe, O., H. Takao, W. Gonoi, H. Sasaki, M. Murakami, H. Kabasawa, H. Kawaguchi, M. Goto, H. Yamada, H. Yamasue, K. Kasai, S. Aoki, and K. Ohtomo. 2010. "Voxel-based analysis of the diffusion tensor." *Neuroradiology* 52 (8):699-710. doi: 10.1007/s00234-010-0716-3.

Adler, J., and I. Parmryd. 2010. "Quantifying colocalization by correlation: the Pearson correlation coefficient is superior to the Mander's overlap coefficient." *Cytometry A* 77 (8):733-42. doi: 10.1002/cyto.a.20896.

Agosta, F., E. Pagani, M. Petrolini, D. Caputo, M. Perini, A. Prelle, F. Salvi, and M. Filippi. 2010. "Assessment of white matter tract damage in patients with amyotrophic lateral sclerosis: a diffusion tensor MR imaging tractography study." *AJNR Am J Neuroradiol* 31 (8):1457-61. doi: 10.3174/ajnr.A2105.

Alba-Ferrara, L. M., and G. A. de Erausquin. 2013. "What does anisotropy measure? Insights from increased and decreased anisotropy in selective fiber tracts in schizophrenia." *Front Integr Neurosci* 7:9. doi: 10.3389/fnint.2013.00009.

Alrafiah, A. R. 2018. "From Mouse Models to Human Disease: An Approach for Amyotrophic Lateral Sclerosis." *In Vivo* 32 (5):983-998. doi: 10.21873/invivo.11339.

Alturkistani, H. A., F. M. Tashkandi, and Z. M. Mohammedsaleh. 2015. "Histological Stains: A Literature Review and Case Study." *Glob J Health Sci* 8 (3):72-9. doi: 10.5539/gjhs.v8n3p72.

Arab, A., A. Wojna-Pelczar, A. Khairnar, N. Szabo, and J. Ruda-Kucerova. 2018. "Principles of diffusion kurtosis imaging and its role in early diagnosis of neurodegenerative disorders." *Brain Res Bull* 139:91-98. doi: 10.1016/j.brainresbull.2018.01.015.

Armstrong, G. A., and P. Drapeau. 2013. "Loss and gain of FUS function impair neuromuscular synaptic transmission in a genetic model of ALS." *Hum Mol Genet* 22 (21):4282-92. doi: 10.1093/hmg/ddt278.

Ash, P. E., Y. J. Zhang, C. M. Roberts, T. Saldi, H. Hutter, E. Buratti, L. Petrucelli, and C. D. Link. 2010. "Neurotoxic effects of TDP-43 overexpression in C. elegans." *Hum Mol Genet* 19 (16):3206-18. doi: 10.1093/hmg/ddq230.

Assaf, Y., T. Blumenfeld-Katzir, Y. Yovel, and P. J. Basser. 2008. "AxCaliber: a method for measuring axon diameter distribution from diffusion MRI." *Magn Reson Med* 59 (6):1347-54. doi: 10.1002/mrm.21577.

Aydogan, D. B., R. Jacobs, S. Dulawa, S. L. Thompson, M. C. Francois, A. W. Toga, H. Dong, J. A. Knowles, and Y. Shi. 2018. "When tractography meets tracer injections: a systematic study of trends and variation sources of diffusion-based connectivity." *Brain Struct Funct* 223 (6):2841-2858. doi: 10.1007/s00429-018-1663-8.

Baloyannis, S. J. 2015a. "Staining neurons with Golgi techniques in degenerative diseases of the brain." *Neural Regen Res* 10 (5):693-5. doi: 10.4103/1673-5374.156950.

Baloyannis, S. J. 2015b. "Staining of dead neurons by the Golgi method in autopsy material." *Methods Mol Biol* 1254:167-79. doi: 10.1007/978-1-4939-2152-2_13.

Barazany, D., P. J. Basser, and Y. Assaf. 2009. "In vivo measurement of axon diameter distribution in the corpus callosum of rat brain." *Brain* 132 (Pt 5):1210-20. doi: 10.1093/brain/awp042.

Barrick, T. R., C. A. Spilling, C. Ingo, J. Madigan, J. D. Isaacs, P. Rich, T. L. Jones, R. L. Magin, M. G. Hall, and F. A. Howe. 2020. "Quasi-diffusion magnetic resonance imaging (QDI): A fast, high b-value diffusion imaging technique." *Neuroimage* 211:116606. doi: 10.1016/j.neuroimage.2020.116606.

Baskoylu, S. N., J. Yersak, P. O'Hern, S. Grosser, J. Simon, S. Kim, K. Schuch, M. Dimitriadi, K. S. Yanagi, J. Lins, and A. C. Hart. 2018. "Single copy/knock-in models of ALS SOD1 in C. elegans suggest loss and gain of function have different contributions to cholinergic and glutamatergic neurodegeneration." *PLoS Genet* 14 (10):e1007682. doi: 10.1371/journal.pgen.1007682.

Basser, P. J., S. Pajevic, C. Pierpaoli, J. Duda, and A. Aldroubi. 2000. "In vivo fiber tractography using DT-MRI data." *Magn Reson Med* 44

(4):625-32. doi: 10.1002/1522-2594(200010)44:4<625::aid-mrm17> 3.0.co;2-o.

Batra, R., and C. W. Lee. 2017. "Mouse Models of C9orf72 Hexanucleotide Repeat Expansion in Amyotrophic Lateral Sclerosis/ Frontotemporal Dementia." *Front Cell Neurosci* 11:196. doi: 10.3389/fncel.2017.00196.

Bennett, K. M., K. M. Schmainda, R. T. Bennett, D. B. Rowe, H. Lu, and J. S. Hyde. 2003. "Characterization of continuously distributed cortical water diffusion rates with a stretched-exponential model." *Magn Reson Med* 50 (4):727-34. doi: 10.1002/mrm.10581.

Bilen, J., and N. M. Bonini. 2005. "Drosophila as a model for human neurodegenerative disease." *Annu Rev Genet* 39:153-71. doi: 10.1146/annurev.genet.39.110304.095804.

Bilican, B., A. Serio, S. J. Barmada, A. L. Nishimura, G. J. Sullivan, M. Carrasco, H. P. Phatnani, C. A. Puddifoot, D. Story, J. Fletcher, I. H. Park, B. A. Friedman, G. Q. Daley, D. J. Wyllie, G. E. Hardingham, I. Wilmut, S. Finkbeiner, T. Maniatis, C. E. Shaw, and S. Chandran. 2012. "Mutant induced pluripotent stem cell lines recapitulate aspects of TDP-43 proteinopathies and reveal cell-specific vulnerability." *Proc Natl Acad Sci U S A* 109 (15):5803-8. doi: 10.1073/pnas.1202922109.

Birger, A., I. Ben-Dor, M. Ottolenghi, T. Turetsky, Y. Gil, S. Sweetat, L. Perez, V. Belzer, N. Casden, D. Steiner, M. Izrael, E. Galun, E. Feldman, O. Behar, and B. Reubinoff. 2019. "Human iPSC-derived astrocytes from ALS patients with mutated C9ORF72 show increased oxidative stress and neurotoxicity." *E Bio Medicine* 50:274-289. doi: 10.1016/j.ebiom.2019.11.026.

Blokhuis, A. M., E. J. Groen, M. Koppers, L. H. van den Berg, and R. J. Pasterkamp. 2013. "Protein aggregation in amyotrophic lateral sclerosis." *Acta Neuropathol* 125 (6):777-94. doi: 10.1007/s00401-013-1125-6.

Bolte, S., and F. P. Cordelieres. 2006. "A guided tour into subcellular colocalization analysis in light microscopy." *J Microsc* 224 (Pt 3):213-32. doi: 10.1111/j.1365-2818.2006.01706.x.

Bontempi, P., A. Busato, R. Bonafede, L. Schiaffino, I. Scambi, A. Sbarbati, R. Mariotti, and P. Marzola. 2018. "MRI reveals therapeutical efficacy of stem cells: An experimental study on the SOD1(G93A) animal model." *Magn Reson Med* 79 (1):459-469. doi: 10.1002/mrm.26685.

Borel, F., G. Gernoux, B. Cardozo, J. P. Metterville, G. C. Toro Cabrera, L. Song, Q. Su, G. P. Gao, M. K. Elmallah, R. H. Brown, Jr., and C. Mueller. 2016. "Therapeutic rAAVrh10 Mediated SOD1 Silencing in Adult SOD1(G93A) Mice and Nonhuman Primates." *Hum Gene Ther* 27 (1):19-31. doi: 10.1089/hum.2015.122.

Borel, F., G. Gernoux, H. Sun, R. Stock, M. Blackwood, R. H. Brown, Jr., and C. Mueller. 2018. "Safe and effective superoxide dismutase 1 silencing using artificial microRNA in macaques." *Sci Transl Med* 10 (465). doi: 10.1126/scitranslmed.aau6414.

Borsodi, F., V. Culea, C. Langkammer, M. Khalil, L. Pirpamer, S. Quasthoff, C. Enzinger, R. Schmidt, F. Fazekas, and S. Ropele. 2017. "Multimodal assessment of white matter tracts in amyotrophic lateral sclerosis." *PLoS One* 12 (6):e0178371. doi: 10.1371/journal.pone.0178371.

Bose, P., G. A. B. Armstrong, and P. Drapeau. 2019. "Neuromuscular junction abnormalities in a zebrafish loss-of-function model of TDP-43." *J Neurophysiol* 121 (1):285-297. doi: 10.1152/jn.00265.2018.

Brenner, D., K. Sieverding, C. Bruno, P. Luningschror, E. Buck, S. Mungwa, L. Fischer, S. J. Brockmann, J. Ulmer, C. Bliederhauser, C. E. Philibert, T. Satoh, S. Akira, S. Boillee, B. Mayer, M. Sendtner, A. C. Ludolph, K. M. Danzer, C. S. Lobsiger, A. Freischmidt, and J. H. Weishaupt. 2019. "Heterozygous Tbk1 loss has opposing effects in early and late stages of ALS in mice." *J Exp Med* 216 (2):267-278. doi: 10.1084/jem.20180729.

Bridge, K. E., N. Berg, R. Adalbert, E. Babetto, T. Dias, M. G. Spillantini, R. R. Ribchester, and M. P. Coleman. 2009. "Late onset distal axonal swelling in YFP-H transgenic mice." *Neurobiol Aging* 30 (2):309-21. doi: 10.1016/j.neurobiolaging.2007.06.002.

Broad, R. J., M. C. Gabel, N. G. Dowell, D. J. Schwartzman, A. K. Seth, H. Zhang, D. C. Alexander, M. Cercignani, and P. N. Leigh. 2019. "Neurite orientation and dispersion density imaging (NODDI) detects cortical and corticospinal tract degeneration in ALS." *J Neurol Neurosurg Psychiatry* 90 (4):404-411. doi: 10.1136/jnnp-2018-318830.

Burk, K., and R. J. Pasterkamp. 2019. "Disrupted neuronal trafficking in amyotrophic lateral sclerosis." *Acta Neuropathol* 137 (6):859-877. doi: 10.1007/s00401-019-01964-7.

Burns, T. C., M. D. Li, S. Mehta, A. J. Awad, and A. A. Morgan. 2015. "Mouse models rarely mimic the transcriptome of human neurodegenerative diseases: A systematic bioinformatics-based critique of preclinical models." *Eur J Pharmacol* 759:101-17. doi: 10.1016/j.ejphar.2015.03.021.

Butti, Z., and S. A. Patten. 2018. "RNA Dysregulation in Amyotrophic Lateral Sclerosis." *Front Genet* 9:712. doi: 10.3389/fgene.2018.00712.

Calabrese, E., A. Badea, G. Cofer, Y. Qi, and G. A. Johnson. 2015. "A Diffusion MRI Tractography Connectome of the Mouse Brain and Comparison with Neuronal Tracer Data." *Cereb Cortex* 25 (11):4628-37. doi: 10.1093/cercor/bhv121.

Cardenas, A. M., J. E. Sarlls, J. Y. Kwan, D. Bageac, Z. S. Gala, L. E. Danielian, A. Ray-Chaudhury, H. W. Wang, K. L. Miller, S. Foxley, S. Jbabdi, R. C. Welsh, and M. K. Floeter. 2017. "Pathology of callosal damage in ALS: An ex-vivo, 7 T diffusion tensor MRI study." *Neuroimage Clin* 15:200-208. doi: 10.1016/j.nicl.2017.04.024.

Carter, Matt, and Jennifer C. Shieh. 2010. *Guide to research techniques in neuroscience*. Amsterdam; Boston: Elsevier/Academic Press.

Carter, Matt, and Jennifer C. Shieh. 2015. *Guide to research techniques in neuroscience*. Second edition. ed. Amsterdam: Elsevier/AP, Academic Press is an imprint of Elsevier.

Casci, I., and U. B. Pandey. 2015. "A fruitful endeavor: modeling ALS in the fruit fly." *Brain Res* 1607:47-74. doi: 10.1016/j.brainres.2014.09.064.

Chadwick, C. S., Entegart Mg Mc, and R. C. Nairn. 1958. "Fluorescent protein tracers; a trial of new fluorochromes and the development of an alternative to fluorescein." *Immunology* 1 (4):315-27.

Chen, G., B. Zhou, H. Zhu, W. Kuang, F. Bi, H. Ai, Z. Gu, X. Huang, S. Lui, and Q. Gong. 2018. "White matter volume loss in amyotrophic lateral sclerosis: A meta-analysis of voxel-based morphometry studies." *Prog Neuropsychopharmacol Biol Psychiatry* 83:110-117. doi: 10.1016/j.pnpbp.2018.01.007.

Chen, H., K. Qian, Z. Du, J. Cao, A. Petersen, H. Liu, L. W. th Blackbourn, C. L. Huang, A. Errigo, Y. Yin, J. Lu, M. Ayala, and S. C. Zhang. 2014. "Modeling ALS with iPSCs reveals that mutant SOD1 misregulates neurofilament balance in motor neurons." *Cell Stem Cell* 14 (6):796-809. doi: 10.1016/j.stem.2014.02.004.

Chen, Z., T. M. Truong, and H. W. Ai. 2017. "Illuminating Brain Activities with Fluorescent Protein-Based Biosensors." *Chemosensors (Basel)* 5 (4). doi: 10.3390/chemosensors5040032.

Chiarotto, G. B., L. P. Cartarozzi, M. Perez, N. P. Biscola, A. B. Spejo, F. Gubert, M. Franca Junior, R. Mendez-Otero, and A. L. R. de Oliveira. 2019. "Tempol improves neuroinflammation and delays motor dysfunction in a mouse model (SOD1(G93A)) of ALS." *J Neuroinflammation* 16 (1):218. doi: 10.1186/s12974-019-1598-x.

Chieppa, M. N., A. Perota, C. Corona, A. Grindatto, I. Lagutina, E. Vallino Costassa, G. Lazzari, S. Colleoni, R. Duchi, F. Lucchini, M. Caramelli, C. Bendotti, C. Galli, and C. Casalone. 2014. "Modeling amyotrophic lateral sclerosis in hSOD1 transgenic swine." *Neurodegener Dis* 13 (4):246-54. doi: 10.1159/000353472.

Chiot, A., C. S. Lobsiger, and S. Boillee. 2019. "New insights on the disease contribution of neuroinflammation in amyotrophic lateral sclerosis." *Curr Opin Neurol* 32 (5):764-770. doi: 10.1097/WCO.0000000000000729.

Choi, Inhee, Elizabeth Lee, and Luke P. Lee. 2014. "Current nano/biotechnological approaches in amyotrophic lateral sclerosis." *Biomedical Engineering Letters* 3 (4):209-222. doi: 10.1007/s13534-013-0114-y.

Chudakov, D. M., M. V. Matz, S. Lukyanov, and K. A. Lukyanov. 2010. "Fluorescent proteins and their applications in imaging living cells and tissues." *Physiol Rev* 90 (3):1103-63. doi: 10.1152/physrev. 00038.2009.

Ciura, S., S. Lattante, I. Le Ber, M. Latouche, H. Tostivint, A. Brice, and E. Kabashi. 2013. "Loss of function of C9orf72 causes motor deficits in a zebrafish model of amyotrophic lateral sclerosis." *Ann Neurol* 74 (2):180-7. doi: 10.1002/ana.23946.

Comi, G., M. Rovaris, and L. Leocani. 1999. "Review neuroimaging in amyotrophic lateral sclerosis." *Eur J Neurol* 6 (6):629-37. doi: 10.1046/j.1468-1331.1999.660629.x.

Cordelieres, F. P., and S. Bolte. 2014. "Experimenters' guide to colocalization studies: finding a way through indicators and quantifiers, in practice." *Methods Cell Biol* 123:395-408. doi: 10.1016/B978-0-12-420138-5.00021-5.

Crivat, G., and J. W. Taraska. 2012. "Imaging proteins inside cells with fluorescent tags." *Trends Biotechnol* 30 (1):8-16. doi: 10.1016/j.tibtech.2011.08.002.

Crociara, P., M. N. Chieppa, E. Vallino Costassa, E. Berrone, M. Gallo, M. Lo Faro, M. D. Pintore, B. Iulini, A. D'Angelo, G. Perona, A. Botter, D. Formicola, A. Rainoldi, M. Paulis, P. Vezzoni, F. Meli, F. A. Peverali, C. Bendotti, M. C. Trolese, L. Pasetto, V. Bonetto, G. Lazzari, R. Duchi, A. Perota, I. Lagutina, C. Quadalti, M. S. Gennero, D. Dezzutto, R. Desiato, M. Boido, M. Ghibaudi, M. C. Valentini, M. Caramelli, C. Galli, C. Casalone, and C. Corona. 2019. "Motor neuron degeneration, severe myopathy and TDP-43 increase in a transgenic pig model of SOD1-linked familiar ALS." *Neurobiol Dis* 124:263-275. doi: 10.1016/j.nbd.2018.11.021.

Cunningham, N. R., B. Kokona, J. M. Quinn, and R. Fairman. 2019. "Size Analysis of C9orf72 Dipeptide Repeat Proteins Expressed in Drosophila melanogaster Using Semidenaturing Detergent Agarose Gel Electrophoresis." *Methods Mol Biol* 2039:91-101. doi: 10.1007/978-1-4939-9678-0_7.

Dadon-Nachum, M., E. Melamed, and D. Offen. 2011. "The "dying-back" phenomenon of motor neurons in ALS." *J Mol Neurosci* 43 (3):470-7. doi: 10.1007/s12031-010-9467-1.

Daducci, A., A. Dal Palu, M. Descoteaux, and J. P. Thiran. 2016. "Microstructure Informed Tractography: Pitfalls and Open Challenges." *Front Neurosci* 10:247. doi: 10.3389/fnins.2016.00247.

Dale, Brian M., Mark A. Brown, Richard C. Semelka, and Mark A. Brown. 2015. *MRI: basic principles and applications*. Fifth edition. ed. Chichester, West Sussex; Hoboken, NJ: John Wiley & Sons, Ltd.

Dantuma, Elise, Stephanie Merchant, and Kiminobu Sugaya. 2010. "Stem cells for the treatment of neurodegenerative diseases." *Stem Cell Research & Therapy* 1 (5):37. doi: 10.1186/scrt37.

Davidson, Michael W., and Mortimer Abramowitz. 2002. "Optical Microscopy." In *Encyclopedia of Imaging Science and Technology*.

Davis, D. A., P. A. Cox, S. A. Banack, P. D. Lecusay, S. P. Garamszegi, M. J. Hagan, J. T. Powell, J. S. Metcalf, R. M. Palmour, A. Beierschmitt, W. G. Bradley, and D. C. Mash. 2020. "l-Serine Reduces Spinal Cord Pathology in a Vervet Model of Preclinical ALS/MND." *J Neuropathol Exp Neurol* 79 (4):393-406. doi: 10.1093/jnen/nlaa002.

De Giorgio, F., C. Maduro, E. M. C. Fisher, and A. Acevedo-Arozena. 2019. "Transgenic and physiological mouse models give insights into different aspects of amyotrophic lateral sclerosis." *Dis Model Mech* 12 (1). doi: 10.1242/dmm.037424.

de Oliveira, G. P., C. J. Alves, and G. Chadi. 2013. "Early gene expression changes in spinal cord from SOD1(G93A) Amyotrophic Lateral Sclerosis animal model." *Front Cell Neurosci* 7:216. doi: 10.3389/fncel.2013.00216.

Di Gregorio, S. E., and M. L. Duennwald. 2018a. "ALS Yeast Models-Past Success Stories and New Opportunities." *Front Mol Neurosci* 11:394. doi: 10.3389/fnmol.2018.00394.

Di Gregorio, S. E., and M. L. Duennwald. 2018b. "Yeast as a model to study protein misfolding in aged cells." *FEMS Yeast Res* 18 (6). doi: 10.1093/femsyr/foy054.

Dietz, M. S., and M. Heilemann. 2019. "Optical super-resolution microscopy unravels the molecular composition of functional protein complexes." *Nanoscale* 11 (39):17981-17991. doi: 10.1039/c9nr06364a.

Dolezalova, D., M. Hruska-Plochan, C. R. Bjarkam, J. C. Sorensen, M. Cunningham, D. Weingarten, J. D. Ciacci, S. Juhas, J. Juhasova, J. Motlik, M. P. Hefferan, T. Hazel, K. Johe, C. Carromeu, A. Muotri, J. Bui, J. Strnadel, and M. Marsala. 2014. "Pig models of neurodegenerative disorders: Utilization in cell replacement-based preclinical safety and efficacy studies." *J Comp Neurol* 522 (12):2784-801. doi: 10.1002/cne.23575.

Donnelly, C. J., P. W. Zhang, J. T. Pham, A. R. Haeusler, N. A. Mistry, S. Vidensky, E. L. Daley, E. M. Poth, B. Hoover, D. M. Fines, N. Maragakis, P. J. Tienari, L. Petrucelli, B. J. Traynor, J. Wang, F. Rigo, C. F. Bennett, S. Blackshaw, R. Sattler, and J. D. Rothstein. 2013. "RNA toxicity from the ALS/FTD C9ORF72 expansion is mitigated by antisense intervention." *Neuron* 80 (2):415-28. doi: 10.1016/j.neuron.2013.10.015.

Draper, A. C. E., Z. Wilson, C. Maile, D. Faccenda, M. Campanella, and R. J. Piercy. 2020. "Species-specific consequences of an E40K missense mutation in superoxide dismutase 1 (SOD1)." *FASEB J* 34 (1):458-473. doi: 10.1096/fj.201901455R.

Duan, W., M. Guo, L. Yi, J. Zhang, Y. Bi, Y. Liu, Y. Li, Z. Li, Y. Ma, G. Zhang, Y. Liu, X. Song, and C. Li. 2019. "Deletion of Tbk1 disrupts autophagy and reproduces behavioral and locomotor symptoms of FTD-ALS in mice." *Aging (Albany NY)* 11 (8):2457-2476. doi: 10.18632/aging.101936.

Dupuis, L., and J. P. Loeffler. 2009. "Neuromuscular junction destruction during amyotrophic lateral sclerosis: insights from transgenic models." *Curr Opin Pharmacol* 9 (3):341-6. doi: 10.1016/j.coph.2009.03.007.

Durand, J., J. Amendola, C. Bories, and B. Lamotte d'Incamps. 2006. "Early abnormalities in transgenic mouse models of amyotrophic lateral sclerosis." *J Physiol Paris* 99 (2-3):211-20. doi: 10.1016/j.jphysparis.2005.12.014.

Endo, Fumito, Okiru Komine, and Koji Yamanaka. 2016. "Neuroinflammation in motor neuron disease." *Clinical and Experimental Neuroimmunology* 7 (2):126-138. doi: 10.1111/cen3.12309.

Ferraiuolo, L., J. Kirby, A. J. Grierson, M. Sendtner, and P. J. Shaw. 2011. "Molecular pathways of motor neuron injury in amyotrophic lateral sclerosis." *Nat Rev Neurol* 7 (11):616-30. doi: 10.1038/nrneurol.2011.152.

Field, A. S., A. Samsonov, A. L. Alexander, P. Mossahebi, and I. D. Duncan. 2019. "Conventional and quantitative MRI in a novel feline model of demyelination and endogenous remyelination." *J Magn Reson Imaging* 49 (5):1304-1311. doi: 10.1002/jmri.26300.

Figley, M. D., and A. D. Gitler. 2013. "Yeast genetic screen reveals novel therapeutic strategy for ALS." *Rare Dis* 1:e24420. doi: 10.4161/rdis.24420.

Fischer, L. R., D. G. Culver, P. Tennant, A. A. Davis, M. Wang, A. Castellano-Sanchez, J. Khan, M. A. Polak, and J. D. Glass. 2004. "Amyotrophic lateral sclerosis is a distal axonopathy: evidence in mice and man." *Exp Neurol* 185 (2):232-40. doi: 10.1016/j.expneurol.2003.10.004.

Fogarty, M. J., P. M. Klenowski, J. D. Lee, J. R. Drieberg-Thompson, S. E. Bartlett, S. T. Ngo, M. A. Hilliard, M. C. Bellingham, and P. G. Noakes. 2016. "Cortical synaptic and dendritic spine abnormalities in a presymptomatic TDP-43 model of amyotrophic lateral sclerosis." *Sci Rep* 6:37968. doi: 10.1038/srep37968.

Fogarty, M. J., E. W. Mu, P. G. Noakes, N. A. Lavidis, and M. C. Bellingham. 2016. "Marked changes in dendritic structure and spine density precede significant neuronal death in vulnerable cortical pyramidal neuron populations in the SOD1(G93A) mouse model of amyotrophic lateral sclerosis." *Acta Neuropathol Commun* 4 (1):77. doi: 10.1186/s40478-016-0347-y.

Fogarty, M. J., P. G. Noakes, and M. C. Bellingham. 2015. "Motor cortex layer V pyramidal neurons exhibit dendritic regression, spine loss, and increased synaptic excitation in the presymptomatic hSOD1(G93A) mouse model of amyotrophic lateral sclerosis." *J Neurosci* 35 (2):643-7. doi: 10.1523/JNEUROSCI.3483-14.2015.

Froeling, Martijn, Pim Pullens, and Alexander Leemans. 2016. "DTI analysis methods: Region of interest analysis." In *Diffusion Tensor Imaging*, 175 - null. Springer New York.

Fujimori, K., M. Ishikawa, A. Otomo, N. Atsuta, R. Nakamura, T. Akiyama, S. Hadano, M. Aoki, H. Saya, G. Sobue, and H. Okano. 2018. "Modeling sporadic ALS in iPSC-derived motor neurons identifies a potential therapeutic agent." *Nat Med* 24 (10):1579-1589. doi: 10.1038/s41591-018-0140-5.

Fujita, K. 2016. "Follow-up review: recent progress in the development of super-resolution optical microscopy." *Microscopy (Oxf)* 65 (4):275-81. doi: 10.1093/jmicro/dfw022.

Fujiyoshi, K., T. Konomi, M. Yamada, K. Hikishima, O. Tsuji, Y. Komaki, S. Momoshima, Y. Toyama, M. Nakamura, and H. Okano. 2013. "Diffusion tensor imaging and tractography of the spinal cord: from experimental studies to clinical application." *Exp Neurol* 242:74-82. doi: 10.1016/j.expneurol.2012.07.015.

Galibert, F., D. Alexandraki, A. Baur, E. Boles, N. Chalwatzis, J. C. Chuat, F. Coster, C. Cziepluch, M. De Haan, H. Domdey, P. Durand, K. D. Entian, M. Gatius, A. Goffeau, L. A. Grivell, A. Hennemann, C. J. Herbert, K. Heumann, F. Hilger, C. P. Hollenberg, M. E. Huang, C. Jacq, J. C. Jauniaux, C. Katsoulou, L. Karpfinger-Hartl, and et al. 1996. "Complete nucleotide sequence of Saccharomyces cerevisiae chromosome X." *EMBO J* 15 (9):2031-49.

Gao, Jin, Mingchen Jiang, Richard L. Magin, Rodolfo G. Gatto, Gerardo Morfini, Andrew C. Larson, and Weiguo Li. 2020. "Multicomponent diffusion analysis reveals microstructural alterations in spinal cord of a mouse model of amyotrophic lateral sclerosis ex vivo." *PLoS One* 15 (4):e0231598. doi: 10.1371/journal.pone.0231598.

Gatto, R., M. Chauhan, and N. Chauhan. 2015. "Anti-edema effects of rhEpo in experimental traumatic brain injury." *Restor Neurol Neurosci* 33 (6):927-41. doi: 10.3233/RNN-150577.

Gatto, R. G. 2018. "Diffusion tensor imaging as a tool to detect presymptomatic axonal degeneration in a preclinical spinal cord model of amyotrophic lateral sclerosis." *Neural Regen Res* 13 (3):425-426. doi: 10.4103/1673-5374.228723.

Gatto, R. G., M. Amin, A. Finkielsztein, C. Weissmann, T. Barrett, C. Lamoutte, O. Uchitel, R. Sumagin, T. H. Mareci, and R. L. Magin. 2019. "Unveiling early cortical and subcortical neuronal degeneration in ALS mice by ultra-high field diffusion MRI." *Amyotroph Lateral Scler Frontotemporal Degener* 20 (7-8):549-561. doi: 10.1080/21678421.2019.1620285.

Gatto, R. G., M. Y. Amin, D. Deyoung, M. Hey, T. H. Mareci, and R. L. Magin. 2018. "Ultra-High Field Diffusion MRI Reveals Early Axonal Pathology in Spinal Cord of ALS mice." *Transl Neurodegener* 7:20. doi: 10.1186/s40035-018-0122-z.

Gatto, R. G., Y. Chu, A. Q. Ye, S. D. Price, E. Tavassoli, A. Buenaventura, S. T. Brady, R. L. Magin, J. H. Kordower, and G. A. Morfini. 2015. "Analysis of YFP(J16)-R6/2 reporter mice and postmortem brains reveals early pathology and increased vulnerability of callosal axons in Huntington's disease." *Hum Mol Genet* 24 (18):5285-98. doi: 10.1093/hmg/ddv248.

Gatto, R. G., W. Li, J. Gao, and R. L. Magin. 2018. "In vivo diffusion MRI detects early spinal cord axonal pathology in a mouse model of amyotrophic lateral sclerosis." *NMR Biomed* 31 (8):e3954. doi: 10.1002/nbm.3954.

Gatto, R. G., W. Li, and R. L. Magin. 2018. "Diffusion tensor imaging identifies presymptomatic axonal degeneration in the spinal cord of ALS mice." *Brain Res* 1679:45-52. doi: 10.1016/j.brainres.2017.11.017.

Gatto, R. G., S. M. Mustafi, M. Y. Amin, T. H. Mareci, Y. C. Wu, and R. L. Magin. 2018. "Neurite orientation dispersion and density imaging can detect presymptomatic axonal degeneration in the spinal cord of ALS mice." *Funct Neurol* 33 (3):155-163.

Gatto, R. G., and C. Weissmann. 2019. "Diffusion Tensor Imaging in Preclinical and Human Studies of Huntington's Disease: What Have we Learned so Far?" *Curr Med Imaging Rev* 15 (6):521-542. doi: 10.2174/1573405614666181115113400.

Gatto, R. G., A. Q. Ye, L. Colon-Perez, T. H. Mareci, A. Lysakowski, S. D. Price, S. T. Brady, M. Karaman, G. Morfini, and R. L. Magin. 2019. "Detection of axonal degeneration in a mouse model of Huntington's disease: comparison between diffusion tensor imaging and anomalous diffusion metrics." *MAGMA* 32 (4):461-471. doi: 10.1007/s10334-019-00742-6.

Gauthier-Kemper, Anne, Carina Weissmann, Hans-Jürgen Reyher, and Roland Brandt. 2012. "Monitoring cytoskeletal dynamics in living neurons using fluorescence photoactivation." *Methods in enzymology* 505:3-21. doi: 10.1016/b978-0-12-388448-0.00009-7.

Genc, B., A. K. Lagrimas, P. Kuru, R. Hess, M. W. Tu, D. M. Menichella, R. J. Miller, A. S. Paller, and P. H. Ozdinler. 2015. "Visualization of Sensory Neurons and Their Projections in an Upper Motor Neuron Reporter Line." *PLoS One* 10 (7):e0132815. doi: 10.1371/journal.pone.0132815.

Genc, B., and P. H. Ozdinler. 2014. "Moving forward in clinical trials for ALS: motor neurons lead the way please." *Drug Discov Today* 19 (4):441-9. doi: 10.1016/j.drudis.2013.10.014.

Gendron, T. F., and L. Petrucelli. 2011. "Rodent models of TDP-43 proteinopathy: investigating the mechanisms of TDP-43-mediated neurodegeneration." *J Mol Neurosci* 45 (3):486-99. doi: 10.1007/s12031-011-9610-7.

Gois, A. M., D. M. F. Mendonca, M. A. M. Freire, and J. R. Santos. 2020. "In Vitro and in Vivo Models of Amyotrophic Lateral Sclerosis: An Updated Overview." *Brain Res Bull* 159:32-43. doi: 10.1016/j.brainresbull.2020.03.012.

Golub, V. M., J. Brewer, X. Wu, R. Kuruba, J. Short, M. Manchi, M. Swonke, I. Younus, and D. S. Reddy. 2015. "Neurostereology protocol for unbiased quantification of neuronal injury and neurodegeneration." *Front Aging Neurosci* 7:196. doi: 10.3389/fnagi.2015.00196.

Gomes, C., C. Escrevente, and J. Costa. 2010. "Mutant superoxide dismutase 1 overexpression in NSC-34 cells: effect of trehalose on aggregation, TDP-43 localization and levels of co-expressed glycoproteins." *Neurosci Lett* 475 (3):145-9. doi: 10.1016/j.neulet. 2010.03.065.

Grenier, K., J. Kao, and P. Diamandis. 2020. "Three-dimensional modeling of human neurodegeneration: brain organoids coming of age." *Mol Psychiatry* 25 (2):254-274. doi: 10.1038/s41380-019-0500-7.

Gurney, M. E. 1994. "Transgenic-mouse model of amyotrophic lateral sclerosis." *N Engl J Med* 331 (25):1721-2. doi: 10.1056/NEJM 199412223312516.

Hajivalili, M., F. Pourgholi, H. S. Kafil, F. Jadidi-Niaragh, and M. Yousefi. 2016. "Mesenchymal Stem Cells in the Treatment of Amyotrophic Lateral Sclerosis." *Curr Stem Cell Res Ther* 11 (1):41-50. doi: 10.2174/1574888x10666150902095031.

Haulcomb, M. M., N. A. Mesnard-Hoaglin, R. J. Batka, R. M. Meadows, W. M. Miller, K. P. McMillan, T. J. Brown, V. M. Sanders, and K. J. Jones. 2015. "Identification of B6SJL mSOD1(G93A) mouse subgroups with different disease progression rates." *J Comp Neurol* 523 (18):2752-68. doi: 10.1002/cne.23814.

Hawrot, J., S. Imhof, and B. J. Wainger. 2020. "Modeling cell-autonomous motor neuron phenotypes in ALS using iPSCs." *Neurobiol Dis* 134:104680. doi: 10.1016/j.nbd.2019.104680.

Hayes, L. R., and J. D. Rothstein. 2016. "C9ORF72-ALS/FTD: Transgenic Mice Make a Come-BAC." *Neuron* 90 (3):427-31. doi: 10.1016/ j.neuron.2016.04.026.

Heiman-Patterson, T. D., J. S. Deitch, E. P. Blankenhorn, K. L. Erwin, M. J. Perreault, B. K. Alexander, N. Byers, I. Toman, and G. M. Alexander. 2005. "Background and gender effects on survival in the TgN(SOD1-G93A)1Gur mouse model of ALS." *J Neurol Sci* 236 (1-2):1-7. doi: 10.1016/j.jns.2005.02.006.

Hirth, F. 2010. "Drosophila melanogaster in the study of human neurodegeneration." *CNS Neurol Disord Drug Targets* 9 (4):504-23. doi: 10.2174/187152710791556104.

Hofling, F., and T. Franosch. 2013. "Anomalous transport in the crowded world of biological cells." *Rep Prog Phys* 76 (4):046602. doi: 10.1088/0034-4885/76/4/046602.

Hogg, M. C., L. Halang, I. Woods, K. S. Coughlan, and J. H. M. Prehn. 2018. "Riluzole does not improve lifespan or motor function in three ALS mouse models." *Amyotroph Lateral Scler Frontotemporal Degener* 19 (5-6):438-445. doi: 10.1080/21678421.2017.1407796.

Holm, I. E., A. K. Alstrup, and Y. Luo. 2016. "Genetically modified pig models for neurodegenerative disorders." *J Pathol* 238 (2):267-87. doi: 10.1002/path.4654.

Huang, C., J. Tong, F. Bi, H. Zhou, and X. G. Xia. 2012. "Mutant TDP-43 in motor neurons promotes the onset and progression of ALS in rats." *J Clin Invest* 122 (1):107-18. doi: 10.1172/JCI59130.

Huang, C., P. Y. Xia, and H. Zhou. 2010. "Sustained expression of TDP-43 and FUS in motor neurons in rodent's lifetime." *Int J Biol Sci* 6 (4):396-406. doi: 10.7150/ijbs.6.396.

Huang, C., H. Zhou, J. Tong, H. Chen, Y. J. Liu, D. Wang, X. Wei, and X. G. Xia. 2011. "FUS transgenic rats develop the phenotypes of amyotrophic lateral sclerosis and frontotemporal lobar degeneration." *PLoS Genet* 7 (3):e1002011. doi: 10.1371/journal.pgen.1002011.

Huang, N. X., Z. Y. Zou, Y. J. Xue, and H. J. Chen. 2020. "Abnormal cerebral microstructures revealed by diffusion kurtosis imaging in amyotrophic lateral sclerosis." *J Magn Reson Imaging* 51 (2):554-562. doi: 10.1002/jmri.26843.

Igaz, L. M., L. K. Kwong, E. B. Lee, A. Chen-Plotkin, E. Swanson, T. Unger, J. Malunda, Y. Xu, M. J. Winton, J. Q. Trojanowski, and V. M. Lee. 2011. "Dysregulation of the ALS-associated gene TDP-43 leads to neuronal death and degeneration in mice." *J Clin Invest* 121 (2):726-38. doi: 10.1172/JCI44867.

Ikenaka, K., Y. Tsukada, A. C. Giles, T. Arai, Y. Nakadera, S. Nakano, K. Kawai, H. Mochizuki, M. Katsuno, G. Sobue, and I. Mori. 2019. "A behavior-based drug screening system using a Caenorhabditis elegans model of motor neuron disease." *Sci Rep* 9 (1):10104. doi: 10.1038/s41598-019-46642-6.

Ito, H. M., Y. Ogura, and M. Tomisaki. 1992. "Stretched-exponential decay laws of general defect diffusion models." *Journal of Statistical Physics* 66 (1-2):563-582. doi: 10.1007/bf01060081.

Jensen, E. C. 2012. "Use of fluorescent probes: their effect on cell biology and limitations." *Anat Rec (Hoboken)* 295 (12):2031-6. doi: 10.1002/ar.22602.

Jensen, J. H., and J. A. Helpern. 2010. "MRI quantification of non-Gaussian water diffusion by kurtosis analysis." *NMR Biomed* 23 (7):698-710. doi: 10.1002/nbm.1518.

Jensen, J. H., J. A. Helpern, A. Ramani, H. Lu, and K. Kaczynski. 2005. "Diffusional kurtosis imaging: the quantification of non-gaussian water diffusion by means of magnetic resonance imaging." *Magn Reson Med* 53 (6):1432-40. doi: 10.1002/mrm.20508.

Jiang, H. Q., M. Ren, H. Z. Jiang, J. Wang, J. Zhang, X. Yin, S. Y. Wang, Y. Qi, X. D. Wang, and H. L. Feng. 2014. "Guanabenz delays the onset of disease symptoms, extends lifespan, improves motor performance and attenuates motor neuron loss in the SOD1 G93A mouse model of amyotrophic lateral sclerosis." *Neuroscience* 277:132-8. doi: 10.1016/j.neuroscience.2014.03.047.

Johansen-Berg, Heidi, and Timothy E. J. Behrens. 2014. *Diffusion MRI: from quantitative measurement to in-vivo neuroanatomy.* 2nd ed. London, UK; Waltham, MA: Elsevier/Academic Press.

Ju, S., D. F. Tardiff, H. Han, K. Divya, Q. Zhong, L. E. Maquat, D. A. Bosco, L. J. Hayward, R. H. Brown, Jr., S. Lindquist, D. Ringe, and G. A. Petsko. 2011. "A yeast model of FUS/TLS-dependent cytotoxicity." *PLoS Biol* 9 (4):e1001052. doi: 10.1371/journal.pbio.1001052.

Julien, J. P., and J. M. Beaulieu. 2000. "Cytoskeletal abnormalities in amyotrophic lateral sclerosis: beneficial or detrimental effects?" *J Neurol Sci* 180 (1-2):7-14. doi: 10.1016/s0022-510x(00)00422-6.

Kamagata, K., T. Hatano, and S. Aoki. 2016. "What is NODDI and what is its role in Parkinson's assessment?" *Expert Rev Neurother* 16 (3):241-3. doi: 10.1586/14737175.2016.1142876.

Kang, S. H., Y. Li, M. Fukaya, I. Lorenzini, D. W. Cleveland, L. W. Ostrow, J. D. Rothstein, and D. E. Bergles. 2013. "Degeneration and impaired regeneration of gray matter oligodendrocytes in amyotrophic lateral sclerosis." *Nat Neurosci* 16 (5):571-9. doi: 10.1038/nn.3357.

Katz, M. L., C. A. Jensen, J. T. Student, G. C. Johnson, and J. R. Coates. 2017. "Cervical spinal cord and motor unit pathology in a canine model of SOD1-associated amyotrophic lateral sclerosis." *J Neurol Sci* 378:193-203. doi: 10.1016/j.jns.2017.05.009.

Keller-Peck, C. R., M. K. Walsh, W. B. Gan, G. Feng, J. R. Sanes, and J. W. Lichtman. 2001. "Asynchronous synapse elimination in neonatal motor units: studies using GFP transgenic mice." *Neuron* 31 (3):381-94. doi: 10.1016/s0896-6273(01)00383-x.

Kingsley, Peter B. 2006. "Introduction to diffusion tensor imaging mathematics: Part I. Tensors, rotations, and eigenvectors." *Concepts in Magnetic Resonance Part A* 28A (2):101-122. doi: 10.1002/cmr.a.20048.

Kino, Y., C. Washizu, M. Kurosawa, M. Yamada, H. Miyazaki, T. Akagi, T. Hashikawa, H. Doi, T. Takumi, G. G. Hicks, N. Hattori, T. Shimogori, and N. Nukina. 2015. "FUS/TLS deficiency causes behavioral and pathological abnormalities distinct from amyotrophic lateral sclerosis." *Acta Neuropathol Commun* 3:24. doi: 10.1186/s40478-015-0202-6.

Kipanyula, M. J., and A. S. Sife. 2018. "Global Trends in Application of Stereology as a Quantitative Tool in Biomedical Research." *Biomed Res Int* 2018:1825697. doi: 10.1155/2018/1825697.

Kobatake, Y., H. Sakai, T. Tsukui, O. Yamato, M. Kohyama, J. Sasaki, S. Kato, M. Urushitani, S. Maeda, and H. Kamishina. 2017. "Localization of a mutant SOD1 protein in E40K-heterozygous dogs: Implications for non-cell-autonomous pathogenesis of degenerative myelopathy." *J Neurol Sci* 372:369-378. doi: 10.1016/j.jns.2016.10.034.

Kobbert, C., R. Apps, I. Bechmann, J. L. Lanciego, J. Mey, and S. Thanos. 2000. "Current concepts in neuroanatomical tracing." *Prog Neurobiol* 62 (4):327-51. doi: 10.1016/s0301-0082(00)00019-8.

Kokona, B., N. R. Cunningham, J. M. Quinn, and R. Fairman. 2019. "Aggregation Profiling of C9orf72 Dipeptide Repeat Proteins Transgenically Expressed in Drosophila melanogaster Using an Analytical Ultracentrifuge Equipped with Fluorescence Detection." *Methods Mol Biol* 2039:81-90. doi: 10.1007/978-1-4939-9678-0_6.

Kremers, Gert-Jan, Sarah G. Gilbert, Paula J. Cranfill, Michael W. Davidson, and David W. Piston. 2011. "Fluorescent proteins at a glance." 124 (2):157-160. doi: 10.1242/jcs.072744% *J Journal of Cell Science*.

Krug, L., N. Chatterjee, R. Borges-Monroy, S. Hearn, W. W. Liao, K. Morrill, L. Prazak, N. Rozhkov, D. Theodorou, M. Hammell, and J. Dubnau. 2017. "Retrotransposon activation contributes to neurodegeneration in a Drosophila TDP-43 model of ALS." *PLoS Genet* 13 (3):e1006635. doi: 10.1371/journal.pgen.1006635.

Kryndushkin, D., and F. Shewmaker. 2011. "Modeling ALS and FTLD proteinopathies in yeast: an efficient approach for studying protein aggregation and toxicity." *Prion* 5 (4):250-7. doi: 10.4161/pri.17229.

Kyrylkova, K., S. Kyryachenko, M. Leid, and C. Kioussi. 2012. "Detection of apoptosis by TUNEL assay." *Methods Mol Biol* 887:41-7. doi: 10.1007/978-1-61779-860-3_5.

Le Bihan, D., J. F. Mangin, C. Poupon, C. A. Clark, S. Pappata, N. Molko, and H. Chabriat. 2001. "Diffusion tensor imaging: concepts and applications." *J Magn Reson Imaging* 13 (4):534-46. doi: 10.1002/jmri.1076.

Lemmens, R., A. Van Hoecke, N. Hersmus, V. Geelen, I. D'Hollander, V. Thijs, L. Van Den Bosch, P. Carmeliet, and W. Robberecht. 2007. "Overexpression of mutant superoxide dismutase 1 causes a motor axonopathy in the zebrafish." *Hum Mol Genet* 16 (19):2359-65. doi: 10.1093/hmg/ddm193.

Lenzi, J., R. De Santis, V. de Turris, M. Morlando, P. Laneve, A. Calvo, V. Caliendo, A. Chio, A. Rosa, and I. Bozzoni. 2015. "ALS mutant FUS proteins are recruited into stress granules in induced pluripotent stem cell-derived motoneurons." *Dis Model Mech* 8 (7):755-66. doi: 10.1242/dmm.020099.

Liachko, N. F., C. R. Guthrie, and B. C. Kraemer. 2010. "Phosphorylation promotes neurotoxicity in a Caenorhabditis elegans model of TDP-43 proteinopathy." *J Neurosci* 30 (48):16208-19. doi: 10.1523/JNEUROSCI.2911-10.2010.

Liang, Yingjie, Allen Q. Ye, Wen Chen, Rodolfo G. Gatto, Luis Colon-Perez, Thomas H. Mareci, and Richard L. Magin. 2016. "A fractal derivative model for the characterization of anomalous diffusion in magnetic resonance imaging." *Communications in Nonlinear Science and Numerical Simulation* 39:529-537. doi: 10.1016/j.cnsns.2016.04.006.

Linares, E., L. V. Seixas, J. N. dos Prazeres, F. V. Ladd, A. A. Ladd, A. A. Coppi, and O. Augusto. 2013. "Tempol moderately extends survival in a hSOD1(G93A) ALS rat model by inhibiting neuronal cell loss, oxidative damage and levels of non-native hSOD1(G93A) forms." *PLoS One* 8 (2):e55868. doi: 10.1371/journal.pone.0055868.

Lipton, Michael L. 2008. *Totally accessible MRI: a user's guide to principles, technology, and applications*. New York; London: Springer.

Liscic, R. M., and D. Breljak. 2011. "Molecular basis of amyotrophic lateral sclerosis." *Prog Neuropsychopharmacol Biol Psychiatry* 35 (2):370-2. doi: 10.1016/j.pnpbp.2010.07.017.

Lissouba, A., M. Liao, E. Kabashi, and P. Drapeau. 2018. "Transcriptomic Analysis of Zebrafish TDP-43 Transgenic Lines." *Front Mol Neurosci* 11 (463):463. doi: 10.3389/fnmol.2018.00463.

Liu, J., and F. Wang. 2017. "Role of Neuroinflammation in Amyotrophic Lateral Sclerosis: Cellular Mechanisms and Therapeutic Implications." *Front Immunol* 8 (1005):1005. doi: 10.3389/fimmu.2017.01005.

Liu, Y., A. Pattamatta, T. Zu, T. Reid, O. Bardhi, D. R. Borchelt, A. T. Yachnis, and L. P. Ranum. 2016. "C9orf72 BAC Mouse Model with Motor Deficits and Neurodegenerative Features of ALS/FTD." *Neuron* 90 (3):521-34. doi: 10.1016/j.neuron.2016.04.005.

Lu, C. H., W. C. Tang, Y. T. Liu, S. W. Chang, F. C. M. Wu, C. Y. Chen, Y. C. Tsai, S. M. Yang, C. W. Kuo, Y. Okada, Y. K. Hwu, P. Chen, and B. C. Chen. 2019. "Lightsheet localization microscopy enables fast, large-scale, and three-dimensional super-resolution imaging." *Commun Biol* 2 (1):177. doi: 10.1038/s42003-019-0403-9.

Lu, J., K. W. Ashwell, R. Hayek, and P. Waite. 2001. "Fluororuby as a marker for detection of acute axonal injury in rat spinal cord." *Brain Res* 915 (1):118-23. doi: 10.1016/s0006-8993(01)02940-7.

Lu, K., C. Q. Vu, T. Matsuda, and T. Nagai. 2019. "Fluorescent Protein-Based Indicators for Functional Super-Resolution Imaging of Biomolecular Activities in Living Cells." *Int J Mol Sci* 20 (22). doi: 10.3390/ijms20225784.

Lu, Y., C. Tang, L. Zhu, J. Li, H. Liang, J. Zhang, and R. Xu. 2016. "The Overexpression of TDP-43 Protein in the Neuron and Oligodendrocyte Cells Causes the Progressive Motor Neuron Degeneration in the SOD1 G93A Transgenic Mouse Model of Amyotrophic Lateral Sclerosis." *Int J Biol Sci* 12 (9):1140-9. doi: 10.7150/ijbs.15938.

Ludolph, A. C. 2013. "Oligodendroglia: new players in amyotrophic lateral sclerosis." *Brain* 136 (Pt 2):370-1. doi: 10.1093/brain/awt017.

Magin, R. L., C. Ingo, L. Colon-Perez, W. Triplett, and T. H. Mareci. 2013. "Characterization of Anomalous Diffusion in Porous Biological Tissues Using Fractional Order Derivatives and Entropy." *Microporous Mesoporous Mater* 178:39-43. doi: 10.1016/j.micromeso.2013.02.054.

Magin, R. L., M. M. Karaman, M. G. Hall, W. Zhu, and X. J. Zhou. 2019. "Capturing complexity of the diffusion-weighted MR signal decay." *Magn Reson Imaging* 56:110-118. doi: 10.1016/j.mri.2018.09.034.

Mancuso, R., S. Olivan, P. Mancera, A. Pasten-Zamorano, R. Manzano, C. Casas, R. Osta, and X. Navarro. 2012. "Effect of genetic background on onset and disease progression in the SOD1-G93A model of amyotrophic lateral sclerosis." *Amyotroph Lateral Scler* 13 (3):302-10. doi: 10.3109/17482968.2012.662688.

Mano, T., A. Albanese, H. U. Dodt, A. Erturk, V. Gradinaru, J. B. Treweek, A. Miyawaki, K. Chung, and H. R. Ueda. 2018. "Whole-Brain Analysis of Cells and Circuits by Tissue Clearing and Light-Sheet Microscopy." *J Neurosci* 38 (44):9330-9337. doi: 10.1523/JNEUROSCI.1677-18.2018.

Mao, Z., S. Zhang, and H. Chen. 2015. "Stem cell therapy for amyotrophic lateral sclerosis." *Cell Regen (Lond)* 4:11. doi: 10.1186/s13619-015-0026-7.

Marconi, S., M. Bonaconsa, I. Scambi, G. M. Squintani, W. Rui, E. Turano, D. Ungaro, S. D'Agostino, F. Barbieri, S. Angiari, A. Farinazzo, G.

Constantin, U. Del Carro, B. Bonetti, and R. Mariotti. 2013. "Systemic treatment with adipose-derived mesenchymal stem cells ameliorates clinical and pathological features in the amyotrophic lateral sclerosis murine model." *Neuroscience* 248:333-43. doi: 10.1016/j.neuroscience.2013.05.034.

McCunn, P., K. M. Gilbert, P. Zeman, A. X. Li, M. J. Strong, A. R. Khan, and R. Bartha. 2019. "Reproducibility of Neurite Orientation Dispersion and Density Imaging (NODDI) in rats at 9.4 Tesla." *PLoS One* 14 (4):e0215974. doi: 10.1371/journal.pone.0215974.

McGown, A., J. R. McDearmid, N. Panagiotaki, H. Tong, S. Al Mashhadi, N. Redhead, A. N. Lyon, C. E. Beattie, P. J. Shaw, and T. M. Ramesh. 2013. "Early interneuron dysfunction in ALS: insights from a mutant sod1 zebrafish model." *Ann Neurol* 73 (2):246-58. doi: 10.1002/ana.23780.

Mead, R. J., E. J. Bennett, A. J. Kennerley, P. Sharp, C. Sunyach, P. Kasher, J. Berwick, B. Pettmann, G. Battaglia, M. Azzouz, A. Grierson, and P. J. Shaw. 2011. "Optimised and rapid pre-clinical screening in the SOD1(G93A) transgenic mouse model of amyotrophic lateral sclerosis (ALS)." *PLoS One* 6 (8):e23244. doi: 10.1371/journal.pone.0023244.

Mina, Maria, Eleni Konsolaki, and Laskaro Zagoraiou. 2018. "Translational Research on Amyotrophic Lateral Sclerosis (ALS): The Preclinical SOD1 Mouse Model." *Journal of Translational Neurosciences* 03 (03). doi: 10.21767/2573-5349.100022.

Mitchell, J. C., P. McGoldrick, C. Vance, T. Hortobagyi, J. Sreedharan, B. Rogelj, E. L. Tudor, B. N. Smith, C. Klasen, C. C. Miller, J. D. Cooper, L. Greensmith, and C. E. Shaw. 2013. "Overexpression of human wild-type FUS causes progressive motor neuron degeneration in an age- and dose-dependent fashion." *Acta Neuropathol* 125 (2):273-88. doi: 10.1007/s00401-012-1043-z.

Miyawaki, A., A. Sawano, and T. Kogure. 2003. "Lighting up cells: labelling proteins with fluorophores." *Nat Cell Biol* Suppl:S1-7.

Morfini, Gerardo, Nadine Schmidt, Carina Weissmann, Gustavo Pigino, and Stefan Kins. 2016. "Conventional kinesin: Biochemical heterogeneity and functional implications in health and disease." *Brain Research Bulletin* 126:347-353. doi: https://doi.org/10.1016/j.brainresbull.2016.06.009.

Mori, S., B. J. Crain, V. P. Chacko, and P. C. van Zijl. 1999. "Three-dimensional tracking of axonal projections in the brain by magnetic resonance imaging." *Ann Neurol* 45 (2):265-9. doi: 10.1002/1531-8249(199902)45:2<265::aid-ana21>3.0.co;2-3.

Morrice, J. R., C. Y. Gregory-Evans, and C. A. Shaw. 2018. "Animal models of amyotrophic lateral sclerosis: A comparison of model validity." *Neural Regen Res* 13 (12):2050-2054. doi: 10.4103/1673-5374.241445.

Moser, B., B. Hochreiter, R. Herbst, and J. A. Schmid. 2017. "Fluorescence colocalization microscopy analysis can be improved by combining object-recognition with pixel-intensity-correlation." *Biotechnol J* 12 (1). doi: 10.1002/biot.201600332.

Moser, J. M., P. Bigini, and T. Schmitt-John. 2013. "The wobbler mouse, an ALS animal model." *Mol Genet Genomics* 288 (5-6):207-29. doi: 10.1007/s00438-013-0741-0.

Moujalled, D., A. Grubman, K. Acevedo, S. Yang, Y. D. Ke, D. M. Moujalled, C. Duncan, A. Caragounis, N. D. Perera, B. J. Turner, M. Prudencio, L. Petrucelli, I. Blair, L. M. Ittner, P. J. Crouch, J. R. Liddell, and A. R. White. 2017. "TDP-43 mutations causing amyotrophic lateral sclerosis are associated with altered expression of RNA-binding protein hnRNP K and affect the Nrf2 antioxidant pathway." *Hum Mol Genet* 26 (9):1732-1746. doi: 10.1093/hmg/ddx093.

Mukherjee, P., S. W. Chung, J. I. Berman, C. P. Hess, and R. G. Henry. 2008. "Diffusion tensor MR imaging and fiber tractography: technical considerations." *AJNR Am J Neuroradiol* 29 (5):843-52. doi: 10.3174/ajnr.A1052.

Mullenbroich, M. C., L. Silvestri, A. P. Di Giovanna, G. Mazzamuto, I. Costantini, L. Sacconi, and F. S. Pavone. 2018. "High-Fidelity Imaging in Brain-Wide Structural Studies Using Light-Sheet Microscopy." *eNeuro* 5 (6). doi: 10.1523/ENEURO.0124-18.2018.

Murakami, T., S. P. Yang, L. Xie, T. Kawano, D. Fu, A. Mukai, C. Bohm, F. Chen, J. Robertson, H. Suzuki, G. G. Tartaglia, M. Vendruscolo, G.

S. Kaminski Schierle, F. T. Chan, A. Moloney, D. Crowther, C. F. Kaminski, M. Zhen, and P. St George-Hyslop. 2012. "ALS mutations in FUS cause neuronal dysfunction and death in Caenorhabditis elegans by a dominant gain-of-function mechanism." *Hum Mol Genet* 21 (1):1-9. doi: 10.1093/hmg/ddr417.

Nardone, R., Y. Holler, A. C. Taylor, P. Lochner, F. Tezzon, S. Golaszewski, F. Brigo, and E. Trinka. 2016. "Canine degenerative myelopathy: a model of human amyotrophic lateral sclerosis." *Zoology (Jena)* 119 (1):64-73. doi: 10.1016/j.zool.2015.09.003.

Nicaise, C., D. Mitrecic, P. Demetter, R. De Decker, M. Authelet, A. Boom, and R. Pochet. 2009. "Impaired blood-brain and blood-spinal cord barriers in mutant SOD1-linked ALS rat." *Brain Res* 1301:152-62. doi: 10.1016/j.brainres.2009.09.018.

Nicaise, C., M. S. Soyfoo, M. Authelet, R. De Decker, D. Bataveljic, C. Delporte, and R. Pochet. 2009. "Aquaporin-4 overexpression in rat ALS model." *Anat Rec (Hoboken)* 292 (2):207-13. doi: 10.1002/ar.20838.

Niessen, H. G., F. Angenstein, K. Sander, W. S. Kunz, M. Teuchert, A. C. Ludolph, H. J. Heinze, H. Scheich, and S. Vielhaber. 2006. "In vivo quantification of spinal and bulbar motor neuron degeneration in the G93A-SOD1 transgenic mouse model of ALS by T2 relaxation time and apparent diffusion coefficient." *Exp Neurol* 201 (2):293-300. doi: 10.1016/j.expneurol.2006.04.007.

Nolan, M., K. Talbot, and O. Ansorge. 2016. "Pathogenesis of FUS-associated ALS and FTD: insights from rodent models." *Acta Neuropathol Commun* 4 (1):99. doi: 10.1186/s40478-016-0358-8.

Nonneman, A., W. Robberecht, and L. Van Den Bosch. 2014. "The role of oligodendroglial dysfunction in amyotrophic lateral sclerosis." *Neurodegener Dis Manag* 4 (3):223-39. doi: 10.2217/nmt.14.21.

Oakes, J. A., M. C. Davies, and M. O. Collins. 2017. "TBK1: a new player in ALS linking autophagy and neuroinflammation." *Mol Brain* 10 (1):5. doi: 10.1186/s13041-017-0287-x.

Ogawa, M., H. Shidara, K. Oka, M. Kurosawa, N. Nukina, and Y. Furukawa. 2015. "Cysteine residues in Cu, Zn-superoxide dismutase are essential to toxicity in Caenorhabditis elegans model of amyotrophic lateral sclerosis." *Biochem Biophys Res Commun* 463 (4):1196-202. doi: 10.1016/j.bbrc.2015.06.084.

Ogawa, M., K. Uchida, O. Yamato, M. Inaba, M. M. Uddin, and H. Nakayama. 2014. "Neuronal loss and decreased GLT-1 expression observed in the spinal cord of Pembroke Welsh Corgi dogs with canine degenerative myelopathy." *Vet Pathol* 51 (3):591-602. doi: 10.1177/0300985813495899.

Oglesby, E., H. A. Quigley, D. J. Zack, F. E. Cone, M. R. Steinhart, J. Tian, M. E. Pease, and G. Kalesnykas. 2012. "Semi-automated, quantitative analysis of retinal ganglion cell morphology in mice selectively expressing yellow fluorescent protein." *Exp Eye Res* 96 (1):107-15. doi: 10.1016/j.exer.2011.12.013.

Okamoto, K., Y. Mizuno, and Y. Fujita. 2008. "Bunina bodies in amyotrophic lateral sclerosis." *Neuropathology* 28 (2):109-15. doi: 10.1111/j.1440-1789.2007.00873.x.

Oshinbolu, S., R. Shah, G. Finka, M. Molloy, M. Uden, and D. G. Bracewell. 2018. "Evaluation of fluorescent dyes to measure protein aggregation within mammalian cell culture supernatants." *J Chem Technol Biotechnol* 93 (3):909-917. doi: 10.1002/jctb.5519.

Pathak, S., E. Cao, M. C. Davidson, S. Jin, and G. A. Silva. 2006. "Quantum dot applications to neuroscience: new tools for probing neurons and glia." *J Neurosci* 26 (7):1893-5. doi: 10.1523/JNEUROSCI.3847-05.2006.

Pérez-Victoria, F. Javier, Guillermo Abascal-Palacios, Igor Tascón, Andrey Kajava, Javier G. Magadán, Erik P. Pioro, Juan S. Bonifacino, and Aitor Hierro. 2010. "Structural basis for the wobbler mouse neurodegenerative disorder caused by mutation in the Vps54 subunit of the GARP complex." 107 (29):12860-12865. doi: 10.1073/pnas.1004756107% *J Proceedings of the National Academy of Sciences*.

Petrou, P., Y. Gothelf, Z. Argov, M. Gotkine, Y. S. Levy, I. Kassis, A. Vaknin-Dembinsky, T. Ben-Hur, D. Offen, O. Abramsky, E. Melamed, and D. Karussis. 2016. "Safety and Clinical Effects of Mesenchymal Stem Cells Secreting Neurotrophic Factor Transplantation in Patients

With Amyotrophic Lateral Sclerosis: Results of Phase 1/2 and 2a Clinical Trials." *JAMA Neurol* 73 (3):337-44. doi: 10.1001/jamaneurol.2015.4321.

Philips, T., and W. Robberecht. 2011. "Neuroinflammation in amyotrophic lateral sclerosis: role of glial activation in motor neuron disease." *Lancet Neurol* 10 (3):253-63. doi: 10.1016/S1474-4422(11)70015-1.

Philips, T., and J. D. Rothstein. 2015. "Rodent Models of Amyotrophic Lateral Sclerosis." *Curr Protoc Pharmacol* 69:5 67 1-5 67 21. doi: 10.1002/0471141755.ph0567s69.

Poesen, K., M. De Schaepdryver, B. Stubendorff, B. Gille, P. Muckova, S. Wendler, T. Prell, T. M. Ringer, H. Rhode, O. Stevens, K. G. Claeys, G. Couwelier, A. D'Hondt, N. Lamaire, P. Tilkin, D. Van Reijen, S. Gourmaud, N. Fedtke, B. Heiling, M. Rumpel, A. Rodiger, A. Gunkel, O. W. Witte, C. Paquet, R. Vandenberghe, J. Grosskreutz, and P. Van Damme. 2017. "Neurofilament markers for ALS correlate with extent of upper and lower motor neuron disease." *Neurology* 88 (24):2302-2309. doi: 10.1212/WNL.0000000000004029.

Querin, G., M. M. El Mendili, P. Bede, S. Delphine, T. Lenglet, V. Marchand-Pauvert, and P. F. Pradat. 2018. "Multimodal spinal cord MRI offers accurate diagnostic classification in ALS." *J Neurol Neurosurg Psychiatry* 89 (11):1220-1221. doi: 10.1136/jnnp-2017-317214.

Ragagnin, A. M. G., S. Shadfar, M. Vidal, M. S. Jamali, and J. D. Atkin. 2019. "Motor Neuron Susceptibility in ALS/FTD." *Front Neurosci* 13:532. doi: 10.3389/fnins.2019.00532.

Ramesh, T., A. N. Lyon, R. H. Pineda, C. Wang, P. M. Janssen, B. D. Canan, A. H. Burghes, and C. E. Beattie. 2010. "A genetic model of amyotrophic lateral sclerosis in zebrafish displays phenotypic hallmarks of motoneuron disease." *Dis Model Mech* 3 (9-10):652-62. doi: 10.1242/dmm.005538.

Ransohoff, R. M. 2018. "All (animal) models (of neurodegeneration) are wrong. Are they also useful?" *J Exp Med* 215 (12):2955-2958. doi: 10.1084/jem.20182042.

Reas, E. T., D. J. Hagler, Jr., N. S. White, J. M. Kuperman, H. Bartsch, K. Cross, R. Q. Loi, A. R. Balachandra, M. J. Meloy, C. E. Wierenga, D. Galasko, J. B. Brewer, A. M. Dale, and L. K. McEvoy. 2017. "Sensitivity of restriction spectrum imaging to memory and neuropathology in Alzheimer's disease." *Alzheimers Res Ther* 9 (1):55. doi: 10.1186/s13195-017-0281-7.

Richard, J. P., and N. J. Maragakis. 2015. "Induced pluripotent stem cells from ALS patients for disease modeling." *Brain Res* 1607:15-25. doi: 10.1016/j.brainres.2014.09.017.

Richter-Landsberg, Christiane. 2007. *Heat shock proteins in neural cells, Neuroscience intelligence unit*. Austin, Tex. New York: Landes Bioscience; Springer Science+Business Media.

Robinson, R. 2011. "A yeast model for understanding ALS: fast, cheap, and easy to control." *PLoS Biol* 9 (4):e1001053. doi: 10.1371/journal.pbio.1001053.

Rosenthal, S. J., J. C. Chang, O. Kovtun, J. R. McBride, and I. D. Tomlinson. 2011. "Biocompatible quantum dots for biological applications." *Chem Biol* 18 (1):10-24. doi: 10.1016/j.chembiol.2010.11.013.

Saberi, S., J. E. Stauffer, D. J. Schulte, and J. Ravits. 2015. "Neuropathology of Amyotrophic Lateral Sclerosis and Its Variants." *Neurol Clin* 33 (4):855-76. doi: 10.1016/j.ncl.2015.07.012.

Sahin, A., A. Held, K. Bredvik, P. Major, T. M. Achilli, A. G. Kerson, K. Wharton, G. Stilwell, and R. Reenan. 2017. "Human SOD1 ALS Mutations in a Drosophila Knock-In Model Cause Severe Phenotypes and Reveal Dosage-Sensitive Gain- and Loss-of-Function Components." *Genetics* 205 (2):707-723. doi: 10.1534/genetics.116.190850.

Sakowski, S. A., J. S. Lunn, A. S. Busta, S. S. Oh, G. Zamora-Berridi, M. Palmer, A. A. Rosenberg, S. G. Philip, J. J. Dowling, and E. L. Feldman. 2012. "Neuromuscular effects of G93A-SOD1 expression in zebrafish." *Mol Neurodegen* 7:44. doi: 10.1186/1750-1326-7-44.

Sarica, A., A. Cerasa, R. Vasta, P. Perrotta, P. Valentino, G. Mangone, P. H. Guzzi, F. Rocca, M. Nonnis, M. Cannataro, and A. Quattrone. 2014.

"Tractography in amyotrophic lateral sclerosis using a novel probabilistic tool: a study with tract-based reconstruction compared to voxel-based approach." *J Neurosci Methods* 224:79-87. doi: 10.1016/j.jneumeth.2013.12.014.

Sato, K., A. Kerever, K. Kamagata, K. Tsuruta, R. Irie, K. Tagawa, H. Okazawa, E. Arikawa-Hirasawa, N. Nitta, I. Aoki, and S. Aoki. 2017. "Understanding microstructure of the brain by comparison of neurite orientation dispersion and density imaging (NODDI) with transparent mouse brain." *Acta Radiol Open* 6 (4):2058460117703816. doi: 10.1177/2058460117703816.

Schlachetzki, J. C., S. W. Saliba, and A. C. Oliveira. 2013. "Studying neurodegenerative diseases in culture models." *Braz J Psychiatry* 35 Suppl 2:S92-100. doi: 10.1590/1516-4446-2013-1159.

Schmitt-John, T. 2015. "VPS54 and the wobbler mouse." *Front Neurosci* 9:381. doi: 10.3389/fnins.2015.00381.

Schoen, M., J. M. Reichel, M. Demestre, S. Putz, D. Deshpande, C. Proepper, S. Liebau, M. J. Schmeisser, A. C. Ludolph, J. Michaelis, and T. M. Boeckers. 2015. "Super-Resolution Microscopy Reveals Presynaptic Localization of the ALS/FTD Related Protein FUS in Hippocampal Neurons." *Front Cell Neurosci* 9:496. doi: 10.3389/fncel.2015.00496.

Shaw, M. P., A. Higginbottom, A. McGown, L. M. Castelli, E. James, G. M. Hautbergue, P. J. Shaw, and T. M. Ramesh. 2018. "Stable transgenic C9orf72 zebrafish model key aspects of the ALS/FTD phenotype and reveal novel pathological features." *Acta Neuropathol Commun* 6 (1):125. doi: 10.1186/s40478-018-0629-7.

Silva, G. A. 2009. "Chapter 2 - Quantum dot nanotechnologies for neuroimaging." *Prog Brain Res* 180:19-34. doi: 10.1016/S0079-6123(08)80002-7.

Smith, S. M., M. Jenkinson, H. Johansen-Berg, D. Rueckert, T. E. Nichols, C. E. Mackay, K. E. Watkins, O. Ciccarelli, M. Z. Cader, P. M. Matthews, and T. E. Behrens. 2006. "Tract-based spatial statistics: voxelwise analysis of multi-subject diffusion data." *Neuroimage* 31 (4):1487-505. doi: 10.1016/j.neuroimage.2006.02.024.

Soares, J. M., P. Marques, V. Alves, and N. Sousa. 2013. "A hitchhiker's guide to diffusion tensor imaging." *Front Neurosci* 7:31. doi: 10.3389/fnins.2013.00031.

Sowa, P., H. F. Harbo, N. S. White, E. G. Celius, H. Bartsch, P. Berg-Hansen, S. M. Moen, A. Bjornerud, L. T. Westlye, O. A. Andreassen, A. M. Dale, and M. K. Beyer. 2019. "Restriction spectrum imaging of white matter and its relation to neurological disability in multiple sclerosis." *Mult Scler* 25 (5):687-698. doi: 10.1177/1352458518 765671.

Sridharan, G., and A. A. Shankar. 2012. "Toluidine blue: A review of its chemistry and clinical utility." *J Oral Maxillofac Pathol* 16 (2):251-5. doi: 10.4103/0973-029X.99081.

Steyaert, J., W. Scheveneels, J. Vanneste, P. Van Damme, W. Robberecht, P. Callaerts, E. Bogaert, and L. Van Den Bosch. 2018. "FUS-induced neurotoxicity in Drosophila is prevented by downregulating nucleocytoplasmic transport proteins." *Hum Mol Genet* 27 (23):4103-4116. doi: 10.1093/hmg/ddy303.

Stoward, P. J., and J. S. Ploem. 1982. "The histochemical basis of quantitative histology." *J Microsc* 128 (Pt 1):49-56. doi: 10.1111/j.1365-2818.1982.tb00436.x.

Suk, K. 2017. "Human-yeast genetic interaction for disease network: systematic discovery of multiple drug targets." *BMB Rep* 50 (11):535-536. doi: 10.5483/bmbrep.2017.50.11.118.

Sun, Z., Z. Diaz, X. Fang, M. P. Hart, A. Chesi, J. Shorter, and A. D. Gitler. 2011. "Molecular determinants and genetic modifiers of aggregation and toxicity for the ALS disease protein FUS/TLS." *PLoS Biol* 9 (4):e1000614. doi: 10.1371/journal.pbio.1000614.

Swash, M. 2020. "Chitinases, neuroinflammation and biomarkers in ALS." *J Neurol Neurosurg Psychiatry* 91 (4):338. doi: 10.1136/jnnp-2019-322520.

Tabata, R. C., J. M. Wilson, P. Ly, P. Zwiegers, D. Kwok, J. M. Van Kampen, N. Cashman, and C. A. Shaw. 2008. "Chronic exposure to dietary sterol glucosides is neurotoxic to motor neurons and induces an

ALS-PDC phenotype." *Neuromolecular Med* 10 (1):24-39. doi: 10.1007/s12017-007-8020-z.

Tallon, C., K. A. Russell, S. Sakhalkar, N. Andrapallayal, and M. H. Farah. 2016. "Length-dependent axo-terminal degeneration at the neuromuscular synapses of type II muscle in SOD1 mice." *Neuroscience* 312:179-89. doi: 10.1016/j.neuroscience.2015.11.018.

Tang, B. L. 2017. "The use of mesenchymal stem cells (MSCs) for amyotrophic lateral sclerosis (ALS) therapy - a perspective on cell biological mechanisms." *Rev Neurosci* 28 (7):725-738. doi: 10.1515/revneuro-2017-0018.

Theart, R. P., B. Loos, Y. S. L. Powrie, and T. R. Niesler. 2018. "Improved region of interest selection and colocalization analysis in three-dimensional fluorescence microscopy samples using virtual reality." *PLoS One* 13 (8):e0201965. doi: 10.1371/journal.pone.0201965.

Therrien, M., G. A. Rouleau, P. A. Dion, and J. A. Parker. 2013. "Deletion of C9ORF72 results in motor neuron degeneration and stress sensitivity in C. elegans." *PLoS One* 8 (12):e83450. doi: 10.1371/journal.pone.0083450.

Thomas, C., F. Q. Ye, M. O. Irfanoglu, P. Modi, K. S. Saleem, D. A. Leopold, and C. Pierpaoli. 2014. "Anatomical accuracy of brain connections derived from diffusion MRI tractography is inherently limited." *Proc Natl Acad Sci U S A* 111 (46):16574-9. doi: 10.1073/pnas.1405672111.

Thompson, A. G., and M. R. Turner. 2019. "Untangling neuroinflammation in amyotrophic lateral sclerosis." *J Neurol Neurosurg Psychiatry* 90 (12):1303-1304. doi: 10.1136/jnnp-2019-321242.

Thomsen, G. M., G. Gowing, J. Latter, M. Chen, J. P. Vit, K. Staggenborg, P. Avalos, M. Alkaslasi, L. Ferraiuolo, S. Likhite, B. K. Kaspar, and C. N. Svendsen. 2014. "Delayed disease onset and extended survival in the SOD1G93A rat model of amyotrophic lateral sclerosis after suppression of mutant SOD1 in the motor cortex." *J Neurosci* 34 (47):15587-600. doi: 10.1523/JNEUROSCI.2037-14.2014.

Thomsen, G. M., G. Gowing, S. Svendsen, and C. N. Svendsen. 2014. "The past, present and future of stem cell clinical trials for ALS." *Exp Neurol* 262 Pt B:127-37. doi: 10.1016/j.expneurol.2014.02.021.

Thonhoff, J. R., P. M. Jordan, J. R. Karam, B. L. Bassett, and P. Wu. 2007. "Identification of early disease progression in an ALS rat model." *Neurosci Lett* 415 (3):264-8. doi: 10.1016/j.neulet.2007.01.028.

Tokuraku, K., M. Marquardt, and T. Ikezu. 2009. "Real-time imaging and quantification of amyloid-beta peptide aggregates by novel quantum-dot nanoprobes." *PLoS One* 4 (12):e8492. doi: 10.1371/journal.pone.0008492.

Tong, J., C. Huang, F. Bi, Q. Wu, B. Huang, X. Liu, F. Li, H. Zhou, and X. G. Xia. 2013. "Expression of ALS-linked TDP-43 mutant in astrocytes causes non-cell-autonomous motor neuron death in rats." *EMBO J* 32 (13):1917-26. doi: 10.1038/emboj.2013.122.

Torre-Fuentes, L., L. Moreno-Jimenez, V. Pytel, J. A. Matias-Guiu, U. Gomez-Pinedo, and J. Matias-Guiu. 2020. "Experimental models of demyelination and remyelination." *Neurologia* 35 (1):32-39. doi: 10.1016/j.nrl.2017.07.002.

Tournier, J. D., S. Mori, and A. Leemans. 2011. "Diffusion tensor imaging and beyond." *Magn Reson Med* 65 (6):1532-56. doi: 10.1002/mrm.22924.

Tovar, Y. Romo L. B., L. D. Santa-Cruz, and R. Tapia. 2009. "Experimental models for the study of neurodegeneration in amyotrophic lateral sclerosis." *Mol Neurodegener* 4:31. doi: 10.1186/1750-1326-4-31.

Tremblay, E., E. Martineau, and R. Robitaille. 2017. "Opposite Synaptic Alterations at the Neuromuscular Junction in an ALS Mouse Model: When Motor Units Matter." *J Neurosci* 37 (37):8901-8918. doi: 10.1523/JNEUROSCI.3090-16.2017.

Tsang, Y. M., F. Chiong, D. Kuznetsov, E. Kasarskis, and C. Geula. 2000. "Motor neurons are rich in non-phosphorylated neurofilaments: cross-species comparison and alterations in ALS." *Brain Res* 861 (1):45-58. doi: 10.1016/s0006-8993(00)01954-5.

Tsao, W., Y. H. Jeong, S. Lin, J. Ling, D. L. Price, P. M. Chiang, and P. C. Wong. 2012. "Rodent models of TDP-43: recent advances." *Brain Res* 1462:26-39. doi: 10.1016/j.brainres.2012.04.031.

Turner, M. R., R. Bowser, L. Bruijn, L. Dupuis, A. Ludolph, M. McGrath, G. Manfredi, N. Maragakis, R. G. Miller, S. L. Pullman, S. B. Rutkove, P. J. Shaw, J. Shefner, and K. H. Fischbeck. 2013. "Mechanisms, models and biomarkers in amyotrophic lateral sclerosis." *Amyotroph Lateral Scler Frontotemporal Degener* 14 Suppl 1:19-32. doi: 10.3109/21678421.2013.778554.

Turner, M. R., J. Grosskreutz, J. Kassubek, S. Abrahams, F. Agosta, M. Benatar, M. Filippi, L. H. Goldstein, M. van den Heuvel, S. Kalra, D. Lule, B. Mohammadi, and A. L. S. first Neuroimaging Symosium in. 2011. "Towards a neuroimaging biomarker for amyotrophic lateral sclerosis." *Lancet Neurol* 10 (5):400-3. doi: 10.1016/S1474-4422(11)70049-7.

Uchida, A., H. Sasaguri, N. Kimura, M. Tajiri, T. Ohkubo, F. Ono, F. Sakaue, K. Kanai, T. Hirai, T. Sano, K. Shibuya, M. Kobayashi, M. Yamamoto, S. Yokota, T. Kubodera, M. Tomori, K. Sakaki, M. Enomoto, Y. Hirai, J. Kumagai, Y. Yasutomi, H. Mochizuki, S. Kuwabara, T. Uchihara, H. Mizusawa, and T. Yokota. 2012. "Non-human primate model of amyotrophic lateral sclerosis with cytoplasmic mislocalization of TDP-43." *Brain* 135 (Pt 3):833-46. doi: 10.1093/brain/awr348.

Van Damme, P., W. Robberecht, and L. Van Den Bosch. 2017. "Modelling amyotrophic lateral sclerosis: progress and possibilities." *Dis Model Mech* 10 (5):537-549. doi: 10.1242/dmm.029058.

Van Hecke, Wim, Wim Van Hecke, Louise Emsell, Stefan Sunaert, and beaux-arts École nationale supérieure des. 2016. *"Diffusion Tensor Imaging: a Practical Handbook."*

van Hummel, A., G. Chan, J. van der Hoven, M. Morsch, S. Ippati, L. Suh, M. Bi, P. R. Asih, W. S. Lee, T. A. Butler, M. Przybyla, G. M. Halliday, O. Piguet, M. C. Kiernan, R. S. Chung, L. M. Ittner, and Y. D. Ke. 2018. "Selective Spatiotemporal Vulnerability of Central Nervous System Neurons to Pathologic TAR DNA-Binding Protein 43 in Aged

Transgenic Mice." *Am J Pathol* 188 (6):1447-1456. doi: 10.1016/j.ajpath.2018.03.002.

Vedantam, A., M. B. Jirjis, B. D. Schmit, M. C. Wang, J. L. Ulmer, and S. N. Kurpad. 2013. "Characterization and limitations of diffusion tensor imaging metrics in the cervical spinal cord in neurologically intact subjects." *J Magn Reson Imaging* 38 (4):861-7. doi: 10.1002/jmri.24039.

Verde, F., V. Silani, and M. Otto. 2019. "Neurochemical biomarkers in amyotrophic lateral sclerosis." *Curr Opin Neurol* 32 (5):747-757. doi: 10.1097/WCO.0000000000000744.

Vijayakumar, U. G., V. Milla, M. Y. Cynthia Stafford, A. J. Bjourson, W. Duddy, and S. M. Duguez. 2019. "A Systematic Review of Suggested Molecular Strata, Biomarkers and Their Tissue Sources in ALS." *Front Neurol* 10:400. doi: 10.3389/fneur.2019.00400.

Vu, L., J. An, T. Kovalik, T. Gendron, L. Petrucelli, and R. Bowser. 2020. "Cross-sectional and longitudinal measures of chitinase proteins in amyotrophic lateral sclerosis and expression of CHI3L1 in activated astrocytes." *J Neurol Neurosurg Psychiatry* 91 (4):350-358. doi: 10.1136/jnnp-2019-321916.

Wang, J., G. W. Farr, D. H. Hall, F. Li, K. Furtak, L. Dreier, and A. L. Horwich. 2009. "An ALS-linked mutant SOD1 produces a locomotor defect associated with aggregation and synaptic dysfunction when expressed in neurons of Caenorhabditis elegans." *PLoS Genet* 5 (1):e1000350. doi: 10.1371/journal.pgen.1000350.

Wang, N., J. Zhang, G. Cofer, Y. Qi, R. J. Anderson, L. E. White, and G. Allan Johnson. 2019. "Neurite orientation dispersion and density imaging of mouse brain microstructure." *Brain Struct Funct* 224 (5):1797-1813. doi: 10.1007/s00429-019-01877-x.

Wang, T., Y. Luo, and G. M. Small. 1994. "The POX1 gene encoding peroxisomal acyl-CoA oxidase in Saccharomyces cerevisiae is under the control of multiple regulatory elements." *J Biol Chem* 269 (39):24480-5.

Wang, X., M. F. Cusick, Y. Wang, P. Sun, J. E. Libbey, K. Trinkaus, R. S. Fujinami, and S. K. Song. 2014. "Diffusion basis spectrum imaging detects and distinguishes coexisting subclinical inflammation, demyelination and axonal injury in experimental autoimmune encephalomyelitis mice." *NMR Biomed* 27 (7):843-52. doi: 10.1002/nbm.3129.

Weissmann, Carina, and Roland Brandt. 2008. "Mechanisms of neurodegenerative diseases: Insights from live cell imaging." 86 (3):504-511. doi: 10.1002/jnr.21448.

Weissmann, Carina, Mariano N. Di Guilmi, Francisco J. Urbano, and Osvaldo D. Uchitel. 2013. "Acute effects of pregabalin on the function and cellular distribution of CaV2.1 in HEK293t cells." *Brain Research Bulletin* 90:107-113. doi: https://doi.org/10.1016/j.brainresbull.2012.10.001.

Welton, T., J. J. Maller, R. M. Lebel, E. T. Tan, D. B. Rowe, and S. M. Grieve. 2019. "Diffusion kurtosis and quantitative susceptibility mapping MRI are sensitive to structural abnormalities in amyotrophic lateral sclerosis." *Neuroimage Clin* 24:101953. doi: 10.1016/j.nicl.2019.101953.

Wen, J., H. Zhang, D. C. Alexander, S. Durrleman, A. Routier, D. Rinaldi, M. Houot, P. Couratier, D. Hannequin, F. Pasquier, J. Zhang, O. Colliot, I. Le Ber, A. Bertrand, Degeneration Predict to Prevent Frontotemporal Lobar, and Group Amyotrophic Lateral Sclerosis Study. 2019. "Neurite density is reduced in the presymptomatic phase of C9orf72 disease." *J Neurol Neurosurg Psychiatry* 90 (4):387-394. doi: 10.1136/jnnp-2018-318994.

Wilson, J. M., I. Khabazian, M. C. Wong, A. Seyedalikhani, J. S. Bains, B. A. Pasqualotto, D. E. Williams, R. J. Andersen, R. J. Simpson, R. Smith, U. K. Craig, L. T. Kurland, and C. A. Shaw. 2002. "Behavioral and neurological correlates of ALS-parkinsonism dementia complex in adult mice fed washed cycad flour." *Neuromolecular Med* 1 (3):207-21. doi: 10.1385/NMM:1:3:207.

Winderickx, J., C. Delay, A. De Vos, H. Klinger, K. Pellens, T. Vanhelmont, F. Van Leuven, and P. Zabrocki. 2008. "Protein folding diseases and neurodegeneration: lessons learned from yeast." *Biochim Biophys Acta* 1783 (7):1381-95. doi: 10.1016/j.bbamcr.2008.01.020.

Winton, M. J., L. M. Igaz, M. M. Wong, L. K. Kwong, J. Q. Trojanowski, and V. M. Lee. 2008. "Disturbance of nuclear and cytoplasmic TAR DNA-binding protein (TDP-43) induces disease-like redistribution, sequestration, and aggregate formation." *J Biol Chem* 283 (19):13302-9. doi: 10.1074/jbc.M800342200.

Wymer, J., and D. R. Borchelt. 2018. "Targeting the Neuromuscular Junction in ALS." *Neurotherapeutics* 15 (3):713-714. doi: 10.1007/s13311-018-0647-y.

Yang, H., G. Wang, H. Sun, R. Shu, T. Liu, C. E. Wang, Z. Liu, Y. Zhao, B. Zhao, Z. Ouyang, D. Yang, J. Huang, Y. Zhou, S. Li, X. Jiang, Z. Xiao, X. J. Li, and L. Lai. 2014. "Species-dependent neuropathology in transgenic SOD1 pigs." *Cell Res* 24 (4):464-81. doi: 10.1038/cr.2014.25.

Zhang, H., T. Schneider, C. A. Wheeler-Kingshott, and D. C. Alexander. 2012. "NODDI: practical in vivo neurite orientation dispersion and density imaging of the human brain." *Neuroimage* 61 (4):1000-16. doi: 10.1016/j.neuroimage.2012.03.072.

Zhang, J., S. Gregory, R. I. Scahill, A. Durr, D. L. Thomas, S. Lehericy, G. Rees, S. J. Tabrizi, H. Zhang, and H. D. investigators TrackOn. 2018. "In vivo characterization of white matter pathology in premanifest huntington's disease." *Ann Neurol* 84 (4):497-504. doi: 10.1002/ana.25309.

Zhang, K., A. N. Coyne, and T. E. Lloyd. 2018. "Drosophila models of amyotrophic lateral sclerosis with defects in RNA metabolism." *Brain Res* 1693 (Pt A):109-120. doi: 10.1016/j.brainres.2018.04.043.

Zhou, H., C. Huang, H. Chen, D. Wang, C. P. Landel, P. Y. Xia, R. Bowser, Y. J. Liu, and X. G. Xia. 2010. "Transgenic rat model of neurodegeneration caused by mutation in the TDP gene." *PLoS Genet* 6 (3):e1000887. doi: 10.1371/journal.pgen.1000887.

BIOGRAPHICAL SKETCHES

Rodolfo Gabriel Gatto, PhD

Affiliation: University of Illinois at Chicago - Department of Bioengineering

Education: University of the Republic, Uruguay (Medical doctor); University of Illinois at Chicago, United States (PhD Bioengineering)

Business Address: University of Illinois at Chicago. Department of Bioengineering. Chicago, IL, US.

Research and Professional Experience: Animal Models, Neuroimaging, Microscopy, Magnetic Resonance Imaging diffusion. Neurodegenerative diseases, Traumatic Brain Injury.

Professional Appointments:

2018-Present: Adjunct Research Assistant Professor. Department of Biomedical Engineering. University of Illinois at Chicago, Chicago, Illinois, USA.

2016-2017: Visiting Research Assistant Professor. Department of Anatomy and Cell Biology. University of Illinois at Chicago, Chicago, Illinois, USA.

2011-2016: Postdoctoral Research Associate. Department of Anatomy and Cell Biology. University of Illinois at Chicago, Chicago, Illinois, USA.

2009-2011: Research Scientist. Research & Development Division, Jesse Brown VA Medical Center. Chicago, Illinois, USA.

2008-2009: Visiting Research Specialist in Health Sciences. Department of Psychiatry, Brain Body Center, University of Illinois at Chicago, Chicago, Illinois, USA.

2004-2007: Visiting Research Specialist in Health Sciences. Department of Neurosurgery, University of Illinois at Chicago, Chicago, Illinois, USA.

Honors & Awards:
2019: Annual Biomedical Research Conference for Minority Students (ABRCMS). Judges' Travel Subsidy award to attend the Annual convention. Anaheim, Convention Center in Anaheim, CA.
2017-2019: National High Field Magnetic Laboratory, Advanced Magnetic Resonance Imaging and Spectroscopy Facility (NHMFL- AMRIS). Magnet Lab Visiting Scientist Program.
2017: Annual Biomedical Research Conference for Minority Students (ABRCMS). Judges' Travel Subsidy award to attend the Annual convention. Phoenix, Convention Center in Phoenix, AZ.
2016: Annual Biomedical Research Conference for Minority Students (ABRCMS). Judges' Travel Subsidy award to attend the Annual convention. Tampa, Convention Center in Tampa, FL.
2016: American Society for Cell Biology Minorities Affairs Committee (ASCB MAC). Travel award to attend Jr. Faculty and Postdoc Career Development Workshop. University of North Carolina, Chapel Hills, NC.
2015: Chicago Biomedical Consortium (CBC). Postdoctoral Research Grant Program. Project Title: "Diffusion Tensor Imaging Analysis as a tool to evaluate axonal pathology in ALS."
2015: Brain Research Foundation (BRF). 15th Annual Neuroscience day (Poster Session Winner) "Addressing the in vivo contribution of JNK3 to Huntington's disease pathogenesis.
2015: College of Medicine Research Forum (COM). University of Illinois at Chicago, Chicago, IL. (Poster Session, Honorable Mention). "The protein kinase JNK3 plays a major role on Huntington's disease pathology."

Publications from the Last 3 Years:
Gatto RG, Weissman C, Amin M, Finkielsztein A, Sumagin R, Mareci TH, Uchitel O. Magin RL (2020). Assessing Neuroaxial Microstructural Changes in a Transgenic Rodent Model of Amyotrophic Lateral Sclerosis by Ultra-High Field MRI and Diffusion Tensor Metrics. *Animal models and Experimental Medicine.* doi:10.1002/ame2.12112.

Gao J, Jiang M, Magin RL, Gatto RG, Morfini G, Larson AC, Li W (2020). Multicomponent Diffusion Analysis of Microstructure Degradation in a Mouse Model of Amyotrophic Lateral Sclerosis (2020). *PloS One.* doi: 10.1371/journal.pone.0231598. [PMID: 32310954].

Gatto RG (2020) Editorial for "Evaluating the Therapeutic Effect of Low-Intensity Transcranial Ultrasound on Traumatic Brain Injury with Diffusion Kurtosis Imaging." *Journal of Magnetic Resonance Imaging.* doi: 10.1002/jmri.27082. [PMID: 32031305].

Gatto RG, Amin M, Finkielsztein A, Weissman C, Barrett T, Lamoutte C, Uchitel O, Sumagin R, Mareci TH and Magin RL (2019). Unveiling Early Cortical and Subcortical Neuronal Degeneration in ALS mice by Ultra-High Field Diffusion MRI. *Journal of Amyotrophic Lateral Sclerosis and Frontotemporal Degeneration.* Jun 3:1-13. 10.1080/21678421.2019.1620285. [PMID: 31159586].

Gatto RG, Ye AQ, Colon-Perez L, Mareci TH, Lysakowski A, Price SD, Brady ST, Morfini GA, Magin RL (2019). Non-invasive detection of callosal axonal degeneration in a mouse model of Huntington's disease: Comparison between diffusion tensor imaging and anomalous diffusion metrics. *Magnetic Resonance Materials in Physics, Biology and Medicine* 10.1007/s10334-019-00742-6. [PMID:30771034].

Gatto RG, Weissmann C (2018). Diffusion Tensor Imaging in Preclinical and Human Studies of Huntington's Disease: What Have we Learned so Far? Current Medical Imaging Reviews Nov; 14(6). doi: 10.2174/1573405614666181115113400.[PMID:32008561].

Gatto RG, Mustafi SM, Amin M, Mareci TH, Wu Yu-Chien and Magin RL (2018). Neurite Orientation Dispersion and Density Imaging can Detect Presymptomatic Axonal Degeneration in the Spinal Cord of ALS mice. *Functional Neurology.* Sept. 33(3):155-163. doi: 10.11138/FNeur/2018.33.3.155. [PMID:30457969].

Gatto RG, Amin M, DeYoung D, Hey M, Mareci TH and Magin RL (2018). Ultra-High Field MRI Diffusion Reveals Early Axonal Pathology in Spinal Cord of ALS mice. *BMC Translational Neurodegeneration,* Aug 8(7); 20. doi: 10.1186/s40035-018-0122-z. [PMID: 30128146].

Gatto RG, Gao J, Li W and Magin RL (2018). *In vivo* Diffusion MRI Detects Early Spinal Cord Axonal Pathology in a Mouse Model of Amyotrophic Lateral Sclerosis. *NMR in Biomedicine,* Aug;31(8): e3954. doi: 10.1002/nbm.3954. [PMID: 30117615].

Gatto RG (2018). Diffusion Tensor Imaging as a Tool to Detect Presymptomatic Axonal Degeneration in a Preclinical Spinal Cord Model of ALS. *Neural Regen Res,* Mar. 13 (3):425-426. [PMID: 29623925].

Gatto RG, Li W and Magin RL. (2018). Diffusion Tensor Imaging Identifies Presymptomatic Axonal Degeneration in the Spinal Cord of ALS Mice. *Brain Research.* Jan. 15 (1679):45-52. [PMID: 29175489].

Carina Weissmann, PhD

Affiliation: IFIBYNE-CONICET (Insituto de Fisiología Biología Molecular y Neurociencias -IFIBYNE-CONICET, University of Buenos Aires, Argentina).

Education: University of Buenos Aires, Argentina (biochemistry degree), University of Osnabrück, Germany (PhD in Neuroscience).

Business Address: IFIBYNE-CONICET, Nuevo edificio, Ciudad Universitaria, CABA 1429, Argentina

Research and Professional Experience: Molecular biology, Cell biology, Biochemistry, Microscopy, Neurodegenerative diseases, cell ion channels.

Professional Appointments:
2019-present: Associate Researcher IFIBYNE-CONICET, Buenos Aires, Argentina
2014-2018: Assisstant Researcher IFIBYNE-CONICET, Buenos Aires, Argentina

2014-2016: Senior Researcher Specialist University of Illinois, Chicago, US.
2014: Invited Assistant Researcher at Loyola Stritch School of Medicine Chicago, US.
2010-2013: Postdoc IFIBYNE-CONICET, Buenos Aires, Argentina.
2009-2010: Postdoc at the VIB Department of Developmental and Molecular Genetics and Department of Human Genetics Katholic University of Leuven (KULeuven), Belgium.

Honors:
2003-2007 PhD in Biology, College 612, University of Osnabrück, Germany. by the DFG (Deutsche Forschung Gemeinschaft).
2012 Travel grant to attend FALAN Neuroscience Congress Cancún, Mexico. by IBRO-LARC.
2014 Shuster Travel award to attend SfN meeting, Washington DC, US. Given by Loyola Stritch School of Medicine.
2017 Special Mention at the Third HD (Huntington's Disease) Contest. Given by Fundación HD Lorena Scarafiocca, Argentina.
2018 Second Prize at the Fourth HD (Huntington's Disease) Contest. Given by Fundación HD Lorena Scarafiocca, Argentina.

Publications from the Last 3 Years:
Gatto RG, Weissman C, Amin M, Finkielsztein A, Sumagin R, Mareci TH, Uchitel O. Magin RL (2020). Assessing Neuraxial Microstructural Changes in a Transgenic Rodent Model of Amyotrophic Lateral Sclerosis by Ultra-High Field MRI and Diffusion Tensor Metrics. *Animal models and Experimental Medicine.* doi:10.1002/ame2.12112.
Uchitel OD, González Inchauspe C, Weissmann C.Synaptic signals mediated by protons and acid-sensing ion channels. *Synapse.* 2019 Oct;73(10).
Gatto RG, Amin M, Finkielsztein A, Weissmann C, Barrett T, Lamoutte C, Uchitel O, Sumagin R, Mareci TH, Magin RL. Unveiling early cortical and subcortical neuronal degeneration in ALS mice by ultra-high field

diffusion MRI. *Amyotroph Lateral Scler Frontotemporal Degener.* 2019 Nov;20(7-8).

Gatto, RG, Weissmann. C. Diffusion Tensor Imaging in Preclinical and Human Studies of Huntington's Disease: What Have we Learned so Far? *Current Medical Imaging* 2018 Volume 15, Issue 6.

Leo L*, Weissmann C*, Burns M*, Kang M, Song Y, Qiang L, Brady ST, Baas PW, Morfini G (*shared first coauthorship). Mutant spastin proteins promote deficits in axonal transport through an isoform-specific mechanism involving casein kinase 2 activation. *Hum Mol Genet.* 2017 Jun 15;26(12):2321-2334.

In: Amyotrophic Lateral Sclerosis
Editor: Julie Sørensen

ISBN: 978-1-53618-193-7
© 2020 Nova Science Publishers, Inc.

Chapter 2

LINGUISTIC PATTERNS IN THE COGNITIVE-AFFECTIVE PROCESSING OF ILLNESS EXPERIENCE: A CASE-CONTROL STUDY OF PATIENTS WITH AMYOTROPHIC LATERAL SCLEROSIS

Andrea Caputo[*]
Department of Dynamic and Clinical Psychology,
"Sapienza" University of Rome, Rome, Italy

ABSTRACT

In recent times, narrative medicine has been developed to recognize, interpret, and make decisions from patients' experiences by focusing on illness-related psychosocial aspects, especially in chronic and rare conditions. With regard to this, research has highlighted the importance of illness stories for the improvement of perceived quality of life among people with Amyotrophic Lateral Sclerosis (ALS). Indeed, therapeutic

---

[*] Corresponding Author's Email: andrea.caputo@uniroma1.it.

writing and expressive disclosure interventions have been demonstrated to facilitate the emotional processing of thoughts and feelings about the ALS experience, with relevant implications for illness adjustment. Based on these premises, the current study aimed at exploring the linguistic patterns in the cognitive-affective processing of illness experience in people with ALS.

To this purpose, a case-control study was conducted on the illness stories of 12 adult Italian patients with ALS (8 women and 4 men), compared to a sample of 12 illness stories of patients (matched by gender) affected by other diverse rare diseases (anorectal atresia, Poland syndrome, and idiopathic pulmonary hypertension). The stories were retrieved through the Internet-based database of the Italian National Centre for Rare Diseases, as part of a community-based participatory project promoted by the Medical Ethics Committee of the Italian National Health Service. Several linguistic measures were inspected, referring to lexical variety (i.e., Average Word Frequency, Type-Token Ratio, and Hapax Percentage), referential activity and semantic specificities. Non-parametric Independent t-tests (Mann-Whitney U) were used to compare indexes of lexical variety and referential activity; whereas, specificity analyses were performed through T-Lab software to compare the vocabularies referring to patients with and without ALS.

The results showed no difference in lexical variety. Instead, with regard to referential activity a higher level of discrepancy between discourse organization and sensory imagery of language ($Mdn = 4$) was found in patients with ALS, compared to patients with other rare diseases ($Mdn = 1.5$), $U = 37.5, p < .05, r = .41$. Besides, some differences emerged that were close to the margin of statistical significance, indicating that narratives of participants with ALS had lower scores of clarity ($Mdn = 4.5$), $U = 39, p = .055, r = -.39$, and discourse organization ($Mdn = 11$), $U = 38.5, p = .052, r = -.40$, than their counterparts ($Mdn = 7$ and $Mdn = 13.5$, respectively). Then, specificity analyses highlighted a higher focus on disease-related impairments, a reduced contextualization of illness into one's life story, and greater efforts to restore a sense of normality in utterances of patients with ALS.

Overall, the present study suggests a biographical disruption caused by illness that threatens self-identity and the quality of symbolization function, as emerging from narratives of patients with ALS compared to those of patients affected by other rare conditions. Narrative medicine could thus benefit from such fruitful insights in order to better understand patients' perspectives, as well as to implement narrative skills in daily practice to enrich general clinical information focused on patients' needs and challenges.

Keywords: amyotrophic lateral sclerosis, illness experience, referential activity, narrative medicine, text analysis

INTRODUCTION

Amyotrophic lateral sclerosis (ALS) represents the most common form of degeneration of motor neurons in adult life and is currently included among rare diseases, with an incidence rate of 2-3 cases per 100,000 person-years, and prevalence of 6-7 per 100,000 across European countries (Logroscino et al., 2009). ALS is a neurodegenerative and chronic condition characterized by several and diverse symptoms, such as fasciculations, paresis, amyotrophy, spasticity (spinal/limb form), swallowing, speaking, and cognitive-behavioral impairments (bulbar form), as well as breathing problems (respiratory form) that may lead to death (Bastos et al., 2011). Given its complex etiology, lack of timely diagnosis and absence of effective treatment (Holtzclaw Williams, 2011), there is an increasing attention to patients' symptom management, care planning and quality of life (Caputo, 2014; Galvin, Gaffney, Corr, Mays, & Hardiman, 2017), highlighting the relevance of perceived health status beyond measures of strength and physical function (Cipolletta, Gammino, & Palmieri, 2017).

In recent times, narrative medicine has been developed to recognize, interpret, and make decisions from patients' experiences by focusing on illness-related psychosocial aspects, especially in chronic and rare conditions (Charon, 2006). This is particularly relevant in the field of ALS (Sakellariou, Boniface, & Brown, 2013), where issues of social isolation, disease-related distress, and family burden are very frequent (Cohen & Biesecker, 2010). Through illness stories (Frank, 1995), patients with ALS can make sense of their experiences and weave them into their lives (Gray, 2009), thus coping with the biographical disruption caused by illness (Caputo, 2013; Locock, Ziebland, & Dumelow, 2009).

Indeed, especially due to the lack of aetiological explanation and decisive treatment of the disease, patients with ALS are confronted with several life challenges threatening their self-identity (Mock & Boerner,

2010), which need to be recognized, accepted and worked through (D'Alberton, Nardi, & Zucchini, 2012). Indeed, the illness narratives of such patients often reveal a high number of psychological implications, such as issues of anxiety, depression, hopelessness and isolation (Caputo, 2014; Diaz et al., 2014; Madsen, Jeppesen, & Handberg, 2018; Sakellariou et al., 2013), that are contrasted by the use of denial and splitting defenses preventing effective psychic elaboration (Brown & Mueller, 1970; Caputo, 2019a).

Concerning this, therapeutic writing and expressive disclosure interventions have been found to facilitate the emotional processing of thoughts and feelings about the ALS experience, with relevant implications for illness adjustment (Harris et al., 2017; Pagnini, Rossi, Lunetta, Banfi, & Corbo, 2010). Indeed, such psychological interventions may contribute to reduce psychological distress and alleviate physical symptoms through promoting emotion regulation and cognitive reframing of negative experiences, which enable the activation of personal resources overall resulting in a better-perceived quality of life (Bryan, LeRoy, & Lu, 2016; Gould et al., 2015; Oberstadt, Esser, Classen, & Mehnert, 2018). As language is considered as a key component of why emotional disclosure is beneficial (Smyth & Pennebaker, 1999), the inspection of some linguistic patterns in patients' writings is, therefore, fruitful to understand the mentalization processes about their illness experience.

Psychic Elaboration and Linguistic Patterns

To grasp the individual's capacity to mentalize experience, several psycholinguistic measures have been developed that can be intended as indicators of cognitive-affective processing, such as lexical variety, referential activity, and semantic specificities.

Lexical variety pertains to the degree of productivity and richness of language, revealing highly differentiated symbolizations as well as greater vitality and flexibility of psychic investment. In this regard, people expressing higher lexical variety are more likely to work on their problems successfully thus getting a better adjustment, compared to those whose verbalizations are more restricted (Page, 1953; Roshal, 1953; Russell, 1987). Instead, verbal redundancy may indicate emotional arousal, confusion and anxiety interrupting the smooth flow of the referential verbal communication, as shown in psychotherapy and counseling research (Chevrie-Muller, Sevestre, & Seguier, 1985; Mowrer, 1953). Indeed, lexical repetitions are associated with a greater difficulty to express an intention or impulse toward action in a linguistic form (e.g., de M'Uzan, 2007; Freud, 1914; Loewald, 1971; Marucco, 2007; Scarfone, 2011). As well, repetitions indicate a reduced integration of contradictory or different affective states, which prevents the creation of new patterns (Halfon & Weinstein, 2013).

Referential activity (RA) refers to the connections between verbal and non-verbal representations (i.e., bodily experience, imagery and affect) (Bucci, Kabasakalian-McKay, & Graham, 2004) in terms of access to sensory experiences and their translation into a linguistic form, based on Bucci's multiple code theory (1997). Therefore, RA allows the recognition, identification, and regulation of emotional states, ensuring a greater sense of control over experience. From such a perspective, higher RA may indicate a better capacity to construct emotional meanings (Bucci, 2007) and encode personal events through language (Sexton & Pennebaker, 2009). Specifically, it provides the basis for affective integration in terms of sensory imagery (i.e., concreteness and imagery) and discourse organization (i.e., specificity and clarity) that can be inferred from the narrator's linguistic style (Bucci, 1997). Consistently, the low levels of RA or the lack of connection between sensory imagery and discourse organization of language may indicate a potential dissociation in emotional processing (Górska, 2013).

Then, by semantic specificities, we mean the specific vocabulary characterizing a given discourse in terms of used lexicon, which enables the exploration of content production to get insights about sense-making processes. The over- or under-used words can suggest subjective meanings in the categorization of personal experience and thus provide clues about emotional and cognitive aspects throughout narratives (Smyth & Pennebaker, 1999). As well, this kind of lexical analysis may allow a better understanding of the elaboration of traumatic experiences and the potential mediating mechanisms within the adjustment process (Baikie & Wilhelm, 2005; Campbell & Pennebaker, 2003; Francis & Pennebaker, 1992; Greenberg et al., 1996; Pennebaker, Chung, Ireland, Gonzales, & Booth, 2007).

From these premises, the current study aimed at exploring the linguistic patterns in the cognitive-affective processing of illness experience in people with ALS, in terms of lexical variety, RA and semantic specificities derived from their illness stories. A case-control study was proposed comparing psycholinguistic measures of patients with ALS with those of patients affected by other diverse rare diseases, to better understand what specifically characterizes the ALS experience and its related psychic elaboration.

METHODS

Participants

The present study comprised illness stories retrieved through the Internet-based database of the Italian National Centre for Rare Diseases, as part of a community-based participatory project promoted by the Medical Ethics Committee of the Italian National Health Service to develop narrative medicine methods at the clinical level in the field of rare diseases. In detail, patients were asked to freely provide an account of their subjective illness experience, with specific regard to their perception of disease and its potential impact on their life. All participants gave their written informed consent to be included in the study before posting their stories.

At the time of research implementation, the illness stories of 12 adult Italian patients with ALS (8 women and 4 men) were present in the database and were all included in the present study. Then, a comparison group was randomly selected from the posted illness stories, referring to 12 patients (matched by gender) that were equally distributed across three different rare diseases, i.e., anorectal atresia (n = 4), Poland syndrome (n = 4), and idiopathic pulmonary hypertension (n = 4). Consistently with the strategy of maximum variation in purposive sampling (Patton, 1987), the comparison group included other rare conditions (affecting less than five in 10,000 citizens in the European Union) featured by a broad diversity of disease etiology and symptoms so to get heterogeneous perspectives. Specifically, anorectal atresia is a congenital defect in which the opening of the anus is absent or misplaced, usually fistulizing anteriorly to the perineum or genitourinary tract. Poland syndrome is marked by a unilateral absence or hypoplasia of the pectoralis major muscle, and a variable degree of ipsilateral hand anomalies, including symbrachydactyly. Then, idiopathic pulmonary hypertension is a progressive and potentially fatal disease, characterized by elevated pulmonary arterial resistance leading to right heart failure.

The sample size of 24 was deemed adequate for studies based on textual material (Vasileiou, Barnett, Thorpe, & Young, 2018), in terms of thematic saturation (Corbin & Strauss, 2008) and information power (Malterud, Siersma, & Guassora, 2016). Textual data from the collected illness stories overall included 18,212 word occurrences, with a mean of 759 words per story.

Psycholinguistic Measures

From the textual data of the retrieved illness stories, some psycholinguistic measures were derived for each participant, referring to lexical variety, RA and semantic specificities.

Concerning lexical variety, three indicators were calculated: the Average Word Frequency (AWF; the occurrence of each word in a given text) as a measure of word repetitiveness; the Type-Token Ratio (TTR; the ratio of different words or types to total words or tokens in the text) as a measure of lexical richness; and the Hapax Percentage (words that appear only once in a text out of the total words) as a measure of lexical specificity.

As well, the RA method was used (Bucci, Kabasakalian-McKay, & Graham, 2004) to assess the degree to which each participant was able to connect verbal and nonverbal representations, based on four scales: concreteness (perceptual and sensory quality), specificity (degree of detail and information), clarity (organization and focus), and imagery (vividness and effectiveness). Specifically, concreteness and imagery scales reflect the level of sensory imagery expressed in language, whereas clarity and specificity scales reflect discourse organization. The scales were rated from 0 to 10 points by three competent judges, by using each illness story as scoring unit. The interclass correlation coefficient (ICC, Shrout & Fleiss, 1979) was used to estimate judges' interrater agreement and showed good reliability for each rated story, with ICC [95% CI] values of 0.85 [0.80, 0.90] for Concreteness, 0.81 [0.77, 0.85] for Specificity, 0.87 [0.83, 0.91] for Clarity, and 0.79 for Imagery [0.74, 0.84]. Then, further indicators were calculated as follows: RA (average of the four scales) as an overall indicator of symbolization function, CONIM (sum of the Concreteness and Imagery scales) reflecting the level of sensory imagery expressed in language, CLASP (sum of the Clarity and Specificity scales) as a measure of discourse organization, and CLASP/CONIM Δ (difference between CLASP and CONIM as absolute value), regarding the level of discrepancy between discourse organization and sensory imagery of language.

Semantic specificities were derived from a computer-aided text analysis conducted through T-Lab software (Lancia, 2004), as already used in past health-related research (Caputo, 2015; Caputo, Giacchetta, & Langher, 2016). Preliminary preparation of the overall textual corpus, comprising 24 illness stories, was performed consisting of the following steps. First, the examination of multiple words that stand for only one meaning, such as compound words (e.g., occupation level), phrasal verbs (e.g., to take away) and idioms (e.g., with respect of). Second, disambiguation of words to resolve semantic ambiguity in homographic words, for example distinguishing "present" as gift and "present" as time. Third, lemmatization involving the reduction of the corpus words to their respective headwords (i.e., lemmas), which entails that verbal forms are taken back to the base form, nouns to the singular form, and so on. The final step was the identification of the keywords list based on the automatically computed frequency threshold (Lancia, 2004). The keywords allow the grasping of the main semantic traits characterizing illness stories and the exploration of the participants' sense-making processes.

Statistical Analyses

Non-parametric Independent t-tests (Mann-Whitney U) were used to compare indexes of lexical variety (i.e., Average Word Frequency, Type-Token Ratio, and Hapax Percentage) and RA (i.e., Concreteness, Specificity, Clarity, Imagery, AR, CONIM, CLASP, and CLASP/CONIM Δ) between patients with and without ALS. Effect sizes (and relative confidence intervals) were also provided through r statistic (which is the Z value from the test divided by the total number of observations).

With regard to semantic specificities, specificity analysis was conducted through T-Lab software to compare the vocabularies referring to illness stories of patients with and without ALS (using ALS as a partitioning variable). Specificity analysis was performed on the final list of 201 keywords resulting from the preliminary preparation of the textual corpus. This procedure allowed the identification of the typical words that were over- or under-used by participants with ALS (compared to their counterparts) in processing their illness experience. The typical words were detected through the chi-square test (χ^2) with $p < .05$ (one degree of freedom), using Cohen's d (95% CI) for estimating the relative effect size.

RESULTS

In Table 1 descriptive statistics of the study variables are shown, with specific regard to lexical variety and RA measures, with skewness and kurtosis values between -2 and +2 overall indicating an acceptable range to prove normal univariate distribution (George and Mallery, 2010).

As reported in Table 2, the result of non-parametric Independent t-tests (Mann-Whitney U) comparing indexes of lexical variety and RA found no difference in lexical variety. Instead, with regard to RA measures, a statistically significant difference emerged. Specifically, a higher level of discrepancy (CLASP/CONIM Δ) between discourse organization and sensory imagery of language ($Mdn = 4$) was found in patients with ALS, compared to patients with other rare diseases ($Mdn = 1.5$), $U = 37.5, p < .05$,

$r = .41$. Besides, some differences emerged that were close to the margin of statistical significance, indicating that narratives of participants with ALS had lower scores of clarity ($Mdn = 4.5$), $U = 39$, $p = .055$, $r = -.39$, and discourse organization ($Mdn = 11$), $U = 38.5$, $p = .052$, $r = -.40$, than their counterparts ($Mdn = 7$ and $Mdn = 13.5$, respectively).

About semantic specificities (Table 3), the results showed that illness stories of patients with ALS were featured by the overuse of the words "ill," "disease," "sick" and "patient," overall suggesting a disease-focused perspective in terms of related limitations, loss of bodily intactness and consequent psychological burden (e.g., "The ill person suffers from the violence of the disease, an unbearable limitation on enjoying his/her body and relations with the world"; "Sometimes disease is so serious that sick people are not able to react"; "Sick people have to be disciplined and patient, infinitely dependent and passive"). The relevance of the experienced ill condition seems to prevail on support and care received from healthcare providers, as confirmed by the presence of "hospital," "doctor," and "physician" among the specificities for defect (e.g., "I can't forget the kindness of the doctor who telephoned me making an appointment for hospitalization"; "I met many attentive, caring physician with whom I established an excellent relationship"). As well, the semantic specificities "world," "person," "communicate" and "difficulty" seem to indicate the patient perception of abnormalcy, social isolation and loss of identity, especially due to altered speech and mobility functions (e.g., "What is a person if s/he cannot communicate?"; "To communicate makes me feel active and belonging to the current world"; "One remembers with difficulty the past emotions as a normal person"). Notwithstanding this, as highlighted by the overuse of words such as "hope" and "positive," efforts to maintain positive expectations toward the future and continue to live with altered circumstances emerge (e.g., "Now, attached to a breathing tube, I still try to understand what hope can be"; "I don't want to leave any stone unturned, a positive mental attitude can make the difference"). The orientation toward imagining an undefined future, rather than toward recalling past biography, seems to be confirmed by the underuse of "child," "age," "month," "baby," "kid," "remember," "parent," which instead refer to a greater contextualization of illness into one's life story (e.g., "At the age of 3 months I was hospitalized in another hospital"; "I remember that as a child I had to devise a way to perform certain manual tasks"; "Thanks to my parents I grew up serenely like all the other kids").

Table 1. Descriptive statistics of lexical variety and referential activity measures

	Mean	SE	SD	Skewness	Kurtosis
Average Word Frequency	1.91	0.08	0.40	0.82	0.80
Typen Token/Ratio	54.41	2.22	10.89	0.20	-0.38
Hapax Percentage	73.90	0.92	4.49	0.60	0.90
Concreteness	5.13	0.60	2.94	0.00	-1.55
Specificity	6.08	0.49	2.41	-0.03	-1.26
Clarity	5.54	0.49	2.40	0.12	-1.01
Imagery	5.33	0.52	2.53	0.19	-1.20
RA	5.52	0.46	2.23	0.39	-1.01
CONIM	10.46	1.08	5.29	0.11	-1.39
CLASP	11.63	0.91	4.47	0.04	-0.73
CLASP/CONIM Δ	3.17	0.54	2.66	0.66	-0.51

Note: SE = Standard Error, SD = Standard deviation.

Table 2. Results of non-parametric Independent t-tests (Mann-Whitney U) comparing patients with and without ALS based on lexical variety and referential activity measures

	Patients with ALS		Patients without ALS		U	Z	r (95% CI)
	Mean	SD	Mean	SD			
Average Word Frequency	2.00	0.48	1.83	0.32	56.00	-0.92	-0.19 (-0.62, 0.24)
Typen Token/Ratio	52.72	12.42	56.11	9.35	56.00	-0.92	-0.19 (-0.62, 0.24)
Hapax Percentage	73.83	5.45	73.97	3.51	67.00	-0.29	-0.06 (-0.49, 0.37)
Concreteness	4.33	2.84	5.92	2.94	47.00	-1.46	-0.30 (-0.73, 0.12)
Specificity	5.25	2.05	6.92	2.54	43.00	-1.69	-0.35 (-0.79, 0.07)
Clarity	4.58	1.93	6.50	2.50	39.00	-1.92	-0.39 (-0.84, 0.01)
Imagery	4.67	1.97	6.00	2.92	52.00	-1.17	-0.24 (-0.67, 0.18)
RA	4.71	1.57	6.33	2.56	44.00	-1.62	-0.33 (-0.77, 0.08)
CONIM	9.00	4.65	11.92	5.68	50.00	-1.28	-0.26 (-0.69, 0.16)
CLASP	9.83	3.49	13.42	4.76	38.50	-1.94	-0.40 (-0.85, 0.01)
CLASP/CONIM Δ	4.33	2.93	2.00	1.81	37.50*	-2.01	-0.41 (-0.86, -0.01)

Note: * Statistically significant at $p < .05$.

Table 3. Semantic specificities of ALS-related illness stories

Over-used words				
Lemma	χ^2	Subtotal	Total	d (95% CI)
Ill	26.28***	40	45	2.37 (1.46, 3.28)
Disease	12.65***	53	74	0.92 (0.42, 1.42)
Sick	10.85***	14	15	3.23 (1.31, 5.16)
World	9.35**	17	20	1.87 (0.67, 3.08)
Person	8.46**	18	22	1.58 (0.52, 2.64)
Hope	8.46**	18	22	1.58 (0.52, 2.64)
Patient	7.61**	15	18	1.71 (0.50, 2.93)
To communicate	5.92*	13	16	1.53 (0.30, 1.77)
Difficulty	5.10*	12	15	1.44 (0.19, 2.68)
Positive	4.22*	9	11	1.58 (0.07, 3.08)
Under-used words				
Lemma	χ^2	Subtotal	Total	d (95% CI)
Hospital	13.85***	16	17	4.19 (1.99, 6.40)
Doctor	13.46***	18	20	2.87 (1.34, 4.40)
Child	12.30***	19	22	2.25 (0.99, 3.51)
Under-used words				
Physician	8.95**	21	27	1.41 (0.49, 2.33)
Age	8.48**	15	18	1.89 (0.62, 3.16)
Baby	7.88**	18	23	1.44 (0.44, 2.95)
Over-used words				
Kid	6.59*	11	13	2.03 (0.48, 3.58)
Month	6.02*	19	26	1.10 (0.22, 1.97)
To remember	5.95*	14	18	1.41 (0.28, 2.53)
Parent	5.40*	15	20	1.22 (0.19, 2.24)

Note: *** Statistically significant at $p < .001$, ** Statistically significant at $p < .01$, *** Statistically significant at $p < .05$.

DISCUSSION

Concerning the objectives of the present research study, the findings showed that patients with ALS and those affected by other rare diseases were comparable in terms of lexical variety, as the degree of productivity and richness of language in their illness stories. Instead, illness narratives of patients with ALS were characterized by a higher level of discrepancy between discourse organization and sensory imagery with a medium effect size, thus indicating a less integrated symbolization function in processing illness experience. In this regard, previous research studies have shown that patients with ALS are confronted with a somatic disruption in terms of body/mind disconnection, which may engender splitting defenses aimed at removing negative affect to preserve the self (Caputo, 2019a; Ferro, Riefolo, Nesci, & Mazza, 1989). This is in line with other psychodynamic studies in health-related fields, such as diabetes (Marchini et al., 2018; Martino et al., 2019; Martino, Caputo, Bellone, Quattropani, & Vicario, 2020), cancer (Tomai, Lauriola, & Caputo, 2018) or drug addiction (Caputo, 2019b, 2019c). Indeed, due to the progressive decline in physical functioning, patients with ALS tend to perceive a loss of control over their body (Caputo, 2019a; Sakellariou et al., 2013), thus feeling a strong sense of uncertainty, not knowing what aspect of life would be lost next (King, Duke, & O'Connor, 2009). Therefore, based on Bucci's multiple code theory (1997), this result could be explained in terms of a greater difficulty of such patients to access to sensory experiences and translate them into language, mostly due to a reduced sense of control over experience.

Further moderate differences - despite not reaching a statistically significant threshold - highlighted that utterances of patients with ALS had lower clarity and discourse organization compared to their counterparts, thus helping better understand the disconnection found in emotional processing.

As clarity overall reflects the narrator's awareness of the communicative intent of discourse as well as of the listener's perspective (Bucci et al., 2004), reduced perspective-taking abilities could be hypothesized, as found in recent studies suggesting social cognitive deficits as a prominent feature of ALS (e.g., Bora, 2017). This could lead to an altered relationship between the self and the external world (Caputo, 2019a), consistent with previous findings about the distance between patients' and caregivers' perspectives (Foley, Timonen, & Hardiman, 2016; Oh & Kim, 2017). Indeed, feelings of loneliness and social isolation are frequent in narratives of patients with ALS (Madsen et al., 2018) and the relational domain is reported as the most salient psychological resource that needs to be developed (Caputo, 2019a).

Another potential interpretation could rely on the fact that clarity mostly pertains to focus, in terms of well-differentiated frames expressed through narrative, and to transition, as the degree of connection between such frames to make sense of this sequencing (Bucci et al., 2004). The reduced clarity could thus indicate a fuzzy framing of illness-related events, overall resulting in a worse discourse organization throughout the narrative, due to the difficulty to make sense of illness in such patients (Mock & Boerner, 2010). Accordingly, this finding could be explained in terms of a biographical disruption caused by illness (Locock et al., 2009), that threatens self-coherence and continuity over the course of the chronic condition (Harnett & Jönson, 2017), rather than as depending on the severity of social cognitive impairment.

The semantic specificities characterizing ALS-related narratives provide further insights to understand the disconnection in the processing of illness experience of such patients, mostly intertwined with the poor quality of their symbolization function. Deepening sense-making processes in their content production, patients with ALS are found to give more salience to their ill identity. This could indicate a gradual process of personification of ALS as a persecutor working to bring about the death of the subject from within, which becomes the protagonist in the narrative (Caputo, 2019a; Schattner, Shahar, & Abu-shakra, 2008; Shahar & Lerman, 2013), consistently with previous studies reporting high levels of death anxiety in such a chronic condition (Caputo, 2019a; Sakellariou et al., 2013). Besides, the scarce references to support received by medical care providers may be explained in terms of patients' refusal of dependency on health services, as a way to maintain autonomy and identity integration (Bassola et al., 2018; Caputo, 2014, 2019a). Indeed, as also found in the present study, search for identity is expressed by patients with ALS, who show greater efforts to restore a sense of normality compared to patients affected by other rare conditions (Bassola, Sansone, & Lusignani, 2018; Caputo, 2014, 2019a; Lemoignan & Ells, 2010; Sakellariou et al., 2013). Specifically, impaired communication emerges as the most relevant issue from patients' perspective, which may negatively affect their intentional agency and social functioning (Caputo, 2014, 2019a; Cipolletta et al., 2017; Fegg et al., 2010). The search for a meaningful life is also highlighted by an effort to maintain positive future expectations, because of the increasing hopelessness due to the ongoing functional decline of the disease (Caputo, 2014; Paganoni et al., 2017). The utterances of patients with ALS seem thus to express the need to cope with the unexpected and thus to learn to live with the disease-related limitations in the future (Sakellariou et al., 2013). Instead, a reduced contextualization of illness into life story emerges, probably revealing a biographical disruption that prevents patients from making sense of past illness events in light of present concerns (Caputo, 2019a; Harnett & Jönson, 2017; Locock et al., 2009; Sakellariou et al., 2013). Overall, such a biographical disruption threatens self-identity and the quality of symbolization function of patients with ALS, as also reflected by the higher dissociation found in the emotional processing of their illness experience, compared to patients affected by other rare conditions.

The present research findings about the ALS experience should be considered as preliminary, in line with a psychological clinical case study approach (Langher, Caputo, & Martino, 2017), and undoubtedly need further investigation. Indeed, several study limitations should be acknowledged, such as the small sample size that does not provide any generalization and the lack of trans-cultural validity, because the collected data refer only to Italian participants. As well, no causal interrelations can be derived between ALS and the examined psycholinguistic measures, given the lack of a baseline assessment and the cross-sectional nature of the study design. Furthermore, the process of psychic elaboration of ALS experience can be affected by many other variables that are not duly taken into account, referring to patients' characteristics (e.g., age, gender), psychological (e.g., emotion regulation, illness-related adjustment) and medical conditions (e.g., duration and severity of the disease, time since diagnosis), as well as context-related information (e.g., social support, family environment).

However, based on our knowledge, this is the first study examining in depth some psycholinguistic measures regarding the cognitive-affective processing of illness experience from the writings of patients with rare conditions. Besides, despite the huge amount of qualitative research on ALS experience, the present study has the added value of using a mixed approach, integrating different strategies of textual data analysis that can reduce potential social desirability bias (Caputo, 2017a). Overall, some clinical psychological implications can be traced from the present case-control study, with specific regard to therapeutic writing and expressive disclosure interventions. Firstly, the promotion of emotional processing of illness experience in patients with ALS should take into account the cognitive reframing of illness-related events into a wider autobiographical memory (Baddeley, 1992). In such a way, it could be possible to reflect on the disruption caused by the disease and to contrast processes of personification and protagonization of illness in one's narrative, thus preserving the good parts of the self and repairing a defective identity (Marchini et al., 2018; Schattner et al., 2008; Shahar & Lerman, 2013). Secondly, a reflective focus on care relationships could be promoted to strengthen the perceived support from formal and informal systems, preventing a hopelessness position and fostering the capacity to communicate and share. Then, a positive expectation toward the future should be integrated with reconstructing the past, so to ensure biographical continuity and rebuild a life trajectory capturing the complexity of the life course (Mattingly & Garro, 2000), in line with the patient need for normalcy and autonomy. Narrative medicine could thus benefit from such fruitful insights in order to better understand patients' perspectives, as well as to implement narrative skills in daily practice to enrich general clinical information focused on patients' needs and challenges (Caputo, 2017b).

REFERENCES

Baddeley, A. (1992). Working memory. *Science, 255*(5044), 556-559. doi:10.1126/science.1736359.

Baikie, K. A., & Wilhelm, K. (2005). Emotional and physical health benefits of expressive writing. *Advances in psychiatric treatment, 11*(5), 338-346. doi:10.1192/apt.11.5.338.

Bassola, B., Sansone, V. A., & Lusignani, M. (2018). Being Yourself and Thinking About the Future in People With Motor Neuron Disease. *Journal of Neuroscience Nursing, 50*(3), 138-143. doi:10.1097/jnn.0000000000000366.

Bastos, A. F., Orsini, M., Machado, D., Pimentel Mello, M., Nader, S., Silva, J. G., Da Silva Catharino, A. M. (2011). Amyotrophic lateral sclerosis: one or multiple causes? *Neurology International, 3*(1), 4. doi:10.4081/ni.2011.e4.

Bora, E. (2017). Meta-analysis of social cognition in amyotrophic lateral sclerosis. *Cortex, 88*, 1-7. doi:10.1016/j.cortex.2016.11.012.

Brown, W. A., & Mueller, P. S. (1970). Psychological Function in Individuals with Amyotrophic Lateral Sclerosis (ALS). *Psychosomatic Medicine, 32*(2), 141-152. doi:10.1097/00006842-197003000-00002.

Bryan, J. L., LeRoy, A. S., & Lu, Q. (2016). The Stargardt disease experience: An analysis of expressive writing essays about living with a rare eye disease. *New Frontiers in Ophthalmology, 2*(1), 57-62. doi:10.15761/NFO.1000116.

Bucci, W. (1997). *Psychoanalysis and Cognitive Science.* New York, NY: Guilford.

Bucci, W. (2007). The role of bodily experience in emotional organization: New perspectives on the multiple code theory. In F. S. Anderson (Ed.), *Bodies in treatment: The unspoken dimension* (pp. 51-76). Hillsdale, NJ: The Analytic Press, Inc.

Bucci, W., Kabasakalian-McKay, R., & Graham, E. (2004). *Scoring referential activity instructions for use with transcripts of spoken texts* (Unpublished manual). Retrieved from https://drive.google.com/file/d/0B6_VEfojheT1YmE2ZjUxNTgtNjgxYi00NGRjLWJlMzAtMzA4YmUyODNkZDE0/view?hl=en.

Campbell, R. S., & Pennebaker, J. W. (2003). The secret life of pronouns: Flexibility in writing style and physical health. *Psychological Science, 14*, 60-65. doi:10.1111/1467-9280.01419.

Caputo, A. (2013). Health demand in primary care context: What do people think about physicians?. *Psychology, Health & Medicine, 18*(2), 145-154. doi: 10.1080/13548506.2012.687828.

Caputo, A. (2015). Trends of psychology-related research on euthanasia: a qualitative software-based thematic analysis of journal abstracts. *Psychology, health & medicine, 20*(7), 858-869. doi:10.1080/13548506.2014.993405.

Caputo, A. (2017a). Social desirability bias in self-reported well-being measures: Evidence from an online survey. *Universitas Psychologica, 16*(2), 245-255. doi:10.11144/Javeriana.upsy16-2.sdsw.

Caputo, A. (2017b). The Contribution of Psychology to Research on Congenital Anomalies (CAs): Computer-Aided Thematic Analysis of International Scientific Literature. In W. Ramirez (Ed.), *Rare Diseases: Prevalence, Treatment Options and Research Insights*. New York: Nova Science Publishers.

Caputo, A. (2019a). Psychodynamic insights from narratives of people with amyotrophic lateral sclerosis: A qualitative phenomenological study. *Mediterranean Journal of Clinical Psychology, 7*(2). doi:10.6092/2282-1619/2019.7.2009.

Caputo, A. (2019b). Deceptive Dynamics in Drug Addiction and Their Role in Control Beliefs and Health Status Reporting: A Study on People With Substance Use Disorder in Treatment. *Journal of Drug Issues* [Article first published online]. doi: 10.1177/0022042619853299.

Caputo, A. (2019c). The Experience of Therapeutic Community: Emotional and Motivational Dynamics of People with Drug Addiction Following Rehabilitation. *International Journal of Mental Health and Addiction, 17*(1), 151–165. doi: 10.1007/s11469-018-0008-4.

Caputo, A., Giacchetta, A., & Langher, V. (2016). AIDS as social construction: text mining of AIDS-related information in the Italian press. *AIDS care, 28*(9), 1171-1176. doi:10.1080/09540121.2016.1153591.

Caputo, A. (2014). Exploring quality of life in Italian patients with rare disease: a computer-aided content analysis of illness stories. *Psychology, Health & Medicine, 19*(2), 211-221. doi:10.1080/13548506.2013.793372.

Charon, D. (2006). Narrative Medicine: Honoring the Stories of Illness. New York: Oxford University Press.

Chevrie-Muller, C., Sevestre, P., & Seguier, N. (1985). Speech and Psychopathology. *Language and Speech, 28*(1), 57–79. doi: 10.1177/002383098502800104.

Cipolletta, S., Gammino, G. R., & Palmieri, A. (2017). Illness trajectories in patients with amyotrophic lateral sclerosis: How illness progression is related to life narratives and interpersonal relationships. *Journal of Clinical Nursing*, *26*(23-24), 5033-5043. doi:10.1111/jocn.14003.

Cohen, J. S., & Biesecker, B. B. (2010). Quality of life in rare genetic conditions: A systematic review of the literature. *American Journal of Medical Genetics Part A*, *152A*(5), 1136-1156. doi:10.1002/ajmg.a.33380.

Corbin, J., & Strauss, A. (2008). *Basics of qualitative research* (3rd ed.). Thousand Oaks, CA: Sage. doi:10.1177/1094428108324688.

D'Alberton, F., Nardi, L., & Zucchini, S. (2012). The onset of a chronic disease as a traumatic psychic experience: A psychodynamic survey on type 1 diabetes in young patients. *Psychoanalytic Psychotherapy*, *26*(4), 294-307. doi:10.1080/02668734.2012.732103.

De M'Uzan, M. (2007). The same and the identical. 1970. *The Psychoanalytic Quarterly*, *76*, 1205-1220. doi:10.1002/j.2167-4086.2007.tb00302.x.

Díaz, J. L., Sancho, J., Barreto, P., Bañuls, P., Renovell, M., & Servera, E. (2014). Effect of a short-term psychological intervention on the anxiety and depression of amyotrophic lateral sclerosis patients. *Journal of Health Psychology*, *21*(7), 1426-1435. doi:10.1177/1359105314554819.

Fegg, M. J., Kögler, M., Brandstätter, M., Jox, R., Anneser, J., Haarmann-Doetkotte, S., Borasio, G. D. (2010). Meaning in life in patients with amyotrophic lateral sclerosis. *Amyotrophic Lateral Sclerosis*, *11*(5), 469-474. doi:10.3109/17482961003692604.

Ferro, F. M., Riefolo, G., Nesci, D. A., & Mazza, S. (1987). Psychodynamic Aspects in Patients with Amyotrophic Lateral Sclerosis (ALS). *Amyotrophic Lateral Sclerosis*, *209*, 313-316. doi:10.1007/978-1-4684-5302-7_46.

Foley, G., Timonen, V., & Hardiman, O. (2016). "I hate being a burden": The patient perspective on carer burden in amyotrophic lateral sclerosis. *Amyotrophic Lateral Sclerosis and Frontotemporal Degeneration*,

17(5-6), 351-357. doi:10.3109/21678421.2016.1143512.

Francis, M. E., & Pennebaker, J. W. (1992). Putting stress into words: Writing about personal upheavals and health. *American Journal of Health Promotion, 6*, 280-287. doi:10.4278/0890-1171-6.4.280.

Frank, A. (1995). *The wounded story teller. Body, illness, and ethics.* Chicago, IL: The University of Chicago Press.

Freud, S. (1914). Remembering, repeating, and working through. In L. Strachey (Ed. & Trans.), *The standard edition of the complete psychological works of Sigmund Freud* (Vol. 12, pp. 145-156). London: Hogarth Press.

Galvin, M., Gaffney, R., Corr, B., Mays, I., & Hardiman, O. (2017). From first symptoms to diagnosis of amyotrophic lateral sclerosis: perspectives of an Irish informal caregiver cohort—a thematic analysis. *BMJ Open, 7*(3), e014985. doi:10.1136/bmjopen-2016-014985

George, D., & Mallery, M. (2010). *SPSS for Windows Step by Step: A Simple Guide and Reference, 17.0 update* (10th ed.) Boston: Pearson.

Górska, D. (2013). Emotions (un)expressed in words: referential activity in borderline personality disorder. *Acta Neuropsychologica, 11*, 143-160.

Gould, R. L., Coulson, M. C., Brown, R. G., Goldstein, L. H., Al-Chalabi, A., & Howard, R. J. (2015). Psychotherapy and pharmacotherapy interventions to reduce distress or improve well-being in people with amyotrophic lateral sclerosis: A systematic review. *Amyotrophic Lateral Sclerosis and Frontotemporal Degeneration, 16*(5-6), 293-302. doi:10.3109/21678421.2015.1062515.

Gray, J. B. (2009). The power of storytelling: Using narrative in the healthcare context. *Journal of Communication in Healthcare, 2*(3), 258-273. doi:10.1179/cih.2009.2.3.258.

Greenberg, M. A., Wortman, C. B., & Stone, A. A. (1996). Emotional expression and physical health: Revising traumatic memories or fostering self-regulation?. *Journal of personality and social psychology, 71*(3), 588-602. doi:10.1037/0022-3514.71.3.588.

Halfon, S., & Weinstein, L. (2013). From compulsion to structure: An empirical model to study invariant repetition and representation. *Psychoanalytic Psychology, 30*(3), 394-422. doi:10.1037/a0033618.

Harnett, T., & Jönson, H. (2017). "They are different now" – Biographical continuity and disruption in nursing home settings. *Journal of Aging Studies, 42*, 1-8. doi:10.1016/j.jaging.2017.05.003.

Harris, M., Thomas, G., Thomas, M., Cafarella, P., Stocks, A., Greig, J., & McEvoy, R. D. (2017). Supporting wellbeing in motor neurone disease for patients, carers, social networks, and health professionals: A scoping review and synthesis. *Palliative and Supportive Care, 16*(02), 228-237. doi:10.1017/s1478951517000700.

Holtzclaw Williams, P. (2011). Policy framework for rare disease health disparities. *Policy, Politics, & Nursing Practice, 12*, 114–118. doi: 10.1177/1527154411404243.

King, S. J., Duke, M. M., & O'Connor, B. A. (2009). Living with amyotrophic lateral sclerosis/motor neurone disease (ALS/MND): decision-making about 'ongoing change and adaptation'. *Journal of Clinical Nursing, 18*(5), 745-754. doi:10.1111/j.1365-2702.2008.02671.x.

Lancia, F. (2004). *Strumenti per l'analisi dei testi: Introduzione all'uso di T-LAB* [*Tools for text analysis: Introduction to the use of T-LAB*]. Milan, IT: Franco Angeli.

Langher, V., Caputo, A., & Martino, G. (2017). What happened to the clinical approach to case study in psychological research? A clinical psychological analysis of scientific articles in high impact-factor journals. *Mediterranean Journal of Clinical Psychology, 5*(3). doi:10.6092/2282-1619/2017.5.1670.

Lemoignan, J., & Ells, C. (2010). Amyotrophic lateral sclerosis and assisted ventilation: How patients decide. *Palliative and Supportive Care, 8*(02), 207-213. doi:10.1017/s1478951510000027.

Locock, L., Ziebland, S., & Dumelow, C. (2009). Biographical disruption, abruption and repair in the context of Motor Neurone Disease. *Sociology of Health & Illness, 31*(7), 1043-1058. doi:10.1111/j.1467-9566.2009.01176.x.

Loewald, H. (1971). Some considerations on repetition and repetition compulsion. *The International Journal of Psychoanalysis, 52*, 59 -66.

Logroscino, G., Traynor, B. J., Hardiman, O., Chio, A., Mitchell, D., & Swingler, R. J. (2009). Incidence of amyotrophic lateral sclerosis in Europe. *Journal of Neurology, Neurosurgery & Psychiatry, 81*(4), 385-390. doi:10.1136/jnnp.2009.183525.

Madsen, L. S., Jeppesen, J., & Handberg, C. (2018). "Understanding my ALS." Experiences and reflections of persons with amyotrophic lateral sclerosis and relatives on participation in peer group rehabilitation. *Disability and Rehabilitation*, 1-9. doi:10.1080/09638288.2018.1429499.

Malterud, K., Siersman, V. D., & Guassora, A. D. (2016). Sample size in qualitative interview studies: Guided by information power. *Qualitative Health Research, 26*(13), 1753-1760. doi: 10.1177/1049732315617444.

Marchini, F., Caputo, A., Napoli, A., Tan Balonan, J., Martino, G., Nannini, V., & Langher, V. (2018). Chronic Illness as Loss of Good Self: Underlying Mechanisms Affecting Diabetes Adaptation. *Mediterranean Journal of Clinical Psychology, 6*(3), 1-25. doi:10.6092/2282-1619/2018.6.1981.

Martino, G., Bellone, F., Langher, V., Caputo, A., Catalano, A., Quattropani, M. C., & Morabito, N. (2019). Alexithymia and Psychological Distress Affect Perceived Quality of Life in Patients with Type 2 Diabetes Mellitus. *Mediterranean Journal of Clinical Psychology, 7*(3). doi:10.6092/2282-1619/2019.7.2328.

Martino, G., Caputo, A., Bellone, F., Quattropani, M. C., & Vicario, C. M. (2020). Going Beyond the Visible in Type 2 Diabetes Mellitus: Defense Mechanisms and their Associations with Depression and Health-Related Quality of Life. *Frontiers in Psychology.* doi:10.3389/fpsyg.2020.00267.

Marucco, N. C. (2007). Between memory and destiny: Repetition. *The International Journal of Psychoanalysis, 88,* 309 -328. doi:10.1516/G27H-3555-1824-N084.

Mattingly, C., & Garro, L. (Eds.) (2000). *Narrative and the Cultural Construction of Illness and Healing.* Berkeley: University of California Press.

Mock, S., & Boerner, K. (2010). Sense Making and Benefit Finding among Patients with Amyotrophic Lateral Sclerosis and Their Primary Caregivers. *Journal of Health Psychology, 15*(1), 115-121. doi:10.1177/1359105309344897.

Mowrer, O. H. (1953). *Psychotherapy: Theory and research.* Oxford, England: Ronald Press Co.; New York, NY, US: Ronald Press Company.

Oberstadt, M. C., Esser, P., Classen, J., & Mehnert, A. (2018). Alleviation of Psychological Distress and the Improvement of Quality of Life in Patients with Amyotrophic Lateral Sclerosis: Adaptation of a Short-Term Psychotherapeutic Intervention. *Frontiers in Neurology, 9.* doi:10.3389/fneur.2018.00231.

Oh, J., & Kim, J. A. (2017). Supportive care needs of patients with amyotrophic lateral sclerosis/motor neuron disease and their caregivers: A scoping review. *Journal of Clinical Nursing, 26*(23-24), 4129-4152. doi:10.1111/jocn.13945.

Paganoni, S., McDonnell, E., Schoenfeld, D., Yu, H., Deng, J., Atassi, H., & Atassi, N. (2017). Functional decline is associated with hopelessness in amyotrophic lateral sclerosis (ALS). *Journal of Neurology & Neurophysiology, 8*(2), e423. doi: 10.4172/2155-9562.1000423.

Page, H. A. (1953). An assessment and predictive value of certain language measures in psychotherapeutic counseling. In W. U. Snyder (Ed.), *Group report of a program of research in psychotherapy* (pp. 88–93). State College, PA: Pennsylvania State University.

Pagnini, F., Rossi, G., Lunetta, C., Banfi, P., & Corbo, M. (2010). Clinical Psychology and Amyotrophic Lateral Sclerosis. *Frontiers in Psychology, 1,* 33. http://doi.org/10.3389/fpsyg.2010.00033.

Pennebaker, J. W., Chung, C. K., Ireland, M., Gonzales, A, & Booth, R. J. (2007). *The development and psychometric properties of LIWC2007. In LIWC2007 Manual.* Retrieved from http://www.LIWC.net.

Roshal, J. G. (1953). The type-token ratio as a measure of change in behavior variability during psychotherapy. In W. U. Snyder (Ed.), *Group report of a program of research in psychotherapy* (pp. 94–104). State College PA.: Pennsylvania State University.

Russell, R. L. (1987). *Language in psychotherapy: Strategies of discovery.* New York: Plenum.

Sakellariou, D., Boniface, G., & Brown, P. (2013). Experiences of living with motor neurone disease: a review of qualitative research. *Disability and Rehabilitation*, *35*(21), 1765-1773. doi:10.3109/09638288.2012.753118.

Scarfone, D. (2011). Repetition: Between presence and meaning. *Canadian Journal of Psychoanalysis*, 19, 70-86.

Schattner, E., Shahar, G., & Abu-Shakra, M. (2008). "I used to dream of lupus as some sort of creature": Chronic illness as an internal object. *American Journal of Orthopsychiatry*, *78*(4), 466-472. doi:10.1037/a0014392.

Sexton, J. D., & Pennebaker, J. W. (2009). The healing powers of expressive writing. In S. B. Kaufman & J. C. Kaufman (Eds.), *The psychology of creative writing* (pp. 264–274). Cambridge: Cambridge University Press. doi:10.1017/CBO9780511627101.018.

Shahar, G., & Lerman, S. F. (2013). The personification of chronic physical illness: Its role in adjustment and implications for psychotherapy integration. *Journal of Psychotherapy Integration*, *23*(1), 49-58. doi:10.1037/a0030272.

Shrout, P. E., & Fleiss, J. L. (1979). Intraclass correlations: Uses in assessing rater reliability. *Psychological Bulletin,* *86*(2), 420–428. doi:10.1037/0033-2909.86.2.420.

Smyth, J. M., & Pennebaker, J. W. (1999). Sharing one's story: Translating emotional experiences into words as a coping tool. In C. R. Snyder (Ed.), *Coping: The psychology of what works* (pp. 70-89). New York: Oxford University Press.

Tomai, M., & Lauriola, M., & Caputo, A. (2018). Are social support and coping styles differently associated with adjustment to cancer in early and advanced stages?. *Mediterranean Journal of Clinical Psychology, 7*(1). doi: 10.6092/2282-1619/2019.7.19831981.

Vasileiou, K., Barnett, J., Thorpe, S., & Young, T. (2018). Characterising and justifying sample size sufficiency in interview-based studies: systematic analysis of qualitative health research over a 15-year period. *BMC medical research methodology, 18*(1), 148. doi:10.1186/s12874-018-0594-7.

In: Amyotrophic Lateral Sclerosis
Editor: Julie Sørensen

ISBN: 978-1-53618-193-7
© 2020 Nova Science Publishers, Inc.

Chapter 3

SENSORY DENERVATION IN MOTOR NEURON DISEASE

Baris Isak[*]
Department of Neurology/Clinical Neurophysiology,
Marmara University, Istanbul, Turkey

ABSTRACT

Identification of amyotrophic lateral sclerosis (ALS) requires demonstration of denervation in motor fibres while sensory fibres are frequently expected to be spared. However, different aspects of sensory involvement in this disease have been extensively reported by many groups for the last three decades. Unfortunately, both the studies with conflicting results and the catastrophic clinical picture due to motor neuron degeneration placed sensory involvement in a relatively neglected position. Today, studies with a new perspective on sensory network in motor neuron diseases are conducted to understand the true extent and patophysiology of ALS and suggest new potential biomarkers to diagnose this tragic disease.

Keywords: amyotrophic lateral sclerosis, sensory, denervation

---

[*] Corresponding Author's Email: barisisak@gmail.com.

INTRODUCTION

Motor neuron diseases (MND) are a family of rare disorders involving upper (e.g., primary lateral sclerosis), or lower motor neurons (e.g., progressive muscular atrophy), or both (i.e., amyotrophic lateral sclerosis-ALS). ALS is the flagship of these diseases owing to its catastrophic lethal progression and to several celebrities who suffered this disease. Referring to distinctive characteristics, i.e., a combination of amyotrophy and degeneration of lateral corticospinal tracts in spine, the disease was named as ALS. ALS presents with asymmetric weakness and atrophy followed by progressive muscular paralysis of limb and/or bulbar muscles. Inevitably, patients die within several years after the disease onset.

SPREAD OF NEURODEGENERATION IN ALS

For ALS, ubiquitin positive cytoplasmic inclusions composed of several proteins were shown in pathological studies (Nakano et al., 2004, Mackenzie et al., 2007). And, as a candidate biomarker of sporadic ALS, phosphorylated 43 kDa transactive response DNA-binding protein (pTDP-43) is the most abundant one among these proteins. Translocation pTDP-43 aggregates from nucleus to cytoplasms of neurons and oligodendrocytes are considered to play a major part in ALS pathogenesis. pTDP-43 is thought to induce a self-inducing process leading to prion like-propagation including several processes like amplification and conversion of native protein to misfolded protein, and spread of abnormal protein aggregates (Braak et al., 2013). In ALS, motor symptoms and signs are discrete and focal initially, but tend to spread in an outward-radiating manner in horizontal and caudal directions. Concordantly, early lesions emerge mainly in agranular frontal cortex and somatomotor neurons in spine and brain stem (stage 1), spreading gradually to adjacent structures i.e., prefrontal cortex, reticular formation, and parvocellular section of red mucleus in stage 2, prefrontal areas and postcentral sensory gyrus in stage 3, anteromedial temporal lobe and hippocampus in stage 4.

In addition, cytoplasmic pTDP-43 was demonstrted also in spinal and peripheral nervous system (Nishihira et al., 2008; Brettschneider et al., 2014).

Therefore, taking involvement of sensory cortex at a relatively advanced stage of the disease and relatively short survival due to catastrophic motor disability into consideration, it is reasonable to understand why clinicians and neurophysiologists neglected the sensory involvement in ALS for a long period.

SENSORY INVOLVEMENT AS A DIAGNOSTIC PROBLEM IN ALS

In practice, clinicans tend to fall into trap of false negative diagnosis more than false positive diagnosis of ALS (Belsh and Schiffman, 1990; Davenport et al., 1996)., Almost 40% of the patients with ALS were found to be misdaignosed for another disease but not ALS, and 27% of the ALS patients were treated for another disease before the ALS diagnosis was settled (Belsh and Schiffman, 1996).

SENSORY DENERVATION IN DIAGNOSTIC CRITERIA OF ALS

For long years, ALS was commonly accepted to be the disease of only motor neurons but sensory network was considered to be intact for accurate diagnosis (Ertekin 1967; Fincham 1964; Stalberg and Sanders, 1992). Later, a number of studies showed mild abnormalities in sensory fibres of ALS patients (Cornblath et al., 1992; Mondelli et al., 1993; Schulte- Mattler et al., 1999; Isaacs et al., 2007). However, in the revised El Escorial criteria, any change attributable to denervation of sensory fibres was accepted as an exclusion criterion for ALS diagnosis (Brooks et al., 2000). And later, findings of denervation in sensory fibres was not accepted as a consequence of primary denervation process but accepted only in the presence of an identifiable cause for sensory neuropathy in the Awaji criteria (e.g., entrapment neuropathy due to cachexia or polyneuropathy) (de Carvalho et al., 2008). Today in practice, despite the continuation of common sense about sensory involvement, many clinicans do not rule out ALS diagnosis based on the subtle changes found in neurophysiological studies.

INVESTIGATIONS FOCUSED ON SENSORY INVOLVEMENT IN ALS

Different aspects of sensory involvement in ALS have been extensively studied by many groups in the last 30 years. But, the studies with conflicting results and the catastrophic clinical picture of ALS due to motor neuron degeneration positioned sensory involvement in a relatively ignored position. In addition, many researchers focused on a limited section of sensory network using a few number of diagnostic procedures in ALS patients. Therefore, the true extent and pattern of sensory involvement in ALS has been a matter of discussion in the last years.

Here, starting from different sensory fibre types in peripheral nervous system and extending to sensory cortex, major studies addressing different aspects of sensory involvement in ALS will be discussed.

A-Beta Fibres

It has long been accepted that sensory nerve conduction studies (NCS) should never be affected in ALS (Ertekin 1967; Fincham 1964; Stalberg and Sanders, 1992). And, both neurologists and clinical neurophysiologists have been stuck to this motto for very long years. In practice, clinical neurophysiologists usually tend to accept abnormal sensory NCS or somatosensory evoked potentials (SEP) as indicators of other MND (e.g., Kennedy disease) or ALS mimic disorders (e.g., radiculopathy, immune polyneuropathies, etc.).

So far, based on diagnostic purposes, most of the studies aimed to investigate the degeneration of the thickest sensory fibres, i.e., A-beta fibres. Although, A-beta fibres were shown to be affected, the percentages of the involvement were not high enough to exclude a secondary pathology or contamination by technical problems. In ALS, denervation of A-beta fibres was shown by several investigators that used sensory NCS (e.g., Cornblath et al., 1992; Mondelli et al., 1993; Schulte- Mattler et al., 1999; Isaacs et al., 2007, Pugdahl et al., 2007 and 2008-Table 1) or somatosensory evoked potentials (SEP) (e.g., Cosi et al., 1984; Dasheiff et al., 1985; Bosch et al., 1985; Matheson et al., 1986; Gregory et al., 1993; Ogata et al., 2001; Hamada et al., 2007- Table 2).

Table 1. Studies that used nerve conduction studies

Author, Issue Year	Tests	Major Results
Fincham and Van Allen, 1964	Median and ulnar NCS	No abnormalities in ALS patients.
Ertekin et al., 1967	Median NCS	No abnormalities in ALS patients.
Shefner et al., 1991	Near nerve sural NCS	Decreased sural CV in 50% and reduced SNAP amplitude in 17% of ALS patients.
Cornblath et al., 1992	NCS	Rare abnormalities in NCS in ALS patients.
Mondelli et al., 1993	NCS	Reduced SNAP amp in sural nerve or distal segments of median and ulnar nerves in ALS patients.
Schulte-Mattler et al., 1999	NCS	Decreased median sensory CV in 13% of ALS patients.
Isaacs et al., 2007	NCS	Sensory abnormalities in ALS patients.
Pugdahl et al., 2008	NCS	Mild sensory abnormalities in 17% of ALS patients.
Pugdahl et al., 2007	NCS	Mild sensory abnormalities in 23% of ALS patients.
Isak et al.,2016	Distal (medial plantar and dorsal sural) and conventional NCS	Abnormal conventional and distal sensory NCS in 44.4% and 66.7% of ALS patients, respectively (total 72.2%).

NCS: nerve conduction study, CV: conduction velocity, SNAP: sensory nerve action potential, ALS: amyotrophic lateral sclerosis,

Table 2. Studies on sensory involvement that used cortical evoked potentials

Author, Issue Year	Tests	Major Results
Cosi et al., 1984	SEP	Prolonged N13 latencies in median-SEP, decreased amplitudes of tibial SEP of ALS patients.
Dasheiff et al., 1985	SEP	Abnormal tibial SEPs in ALS patients.
Bosch et al., 1985	SEP	SEPs were abnormal in 57% of the ALS patients. N32 and/or N60 were delayed or absent in ALS patients. Early potentials were intact.
Matheson et al., 1986	VEP, SEP, BAEP, and H-reflexes	59%, 34%, 12%, and 12% of the ALS patients had abnormal median-SEPs, tibial-SEPs, BAEPs, and VEPs respectively.
Gregory et al., 1993	SNAPs, VT	Non-significant increase in VT, significant decrease in SNAP amp, and significant prolongation in SEP-N19 latency of ALS patients.
Ogata et al., 2001	SEP, sensory nerve conduction velocities	25% of the ALS patients had signs of pseudo bulbar palsy and abnormal posterior tibial nerve and/or median nerve SEPs, suggesting a form of clinical subtype.
Hamada et al., 2007	SEP, CCT	Increased SEP amplitudes and prolonged CCT in ALS patients.
Xu et al., 2009	CHEP and SEP	No abnormalities in ALS patients.
Simone et al., 2010	LEP in upper extremities	Prolonged LEP latencies and increased LEP amp in ALS patients.
Isak et al., 2016	LEP and SEP	Abnormal LEPs and SEPs in 72.2% and 56.6% of ALS patients, respectively.

SEP: somatosensory evoked potential, VEP: visual evoked potential, BAEP: brain auditory rvoked potential, SNAP: sensory nerve action potential, VT: vibration threshold, CCT: central conduction time, CHEP: contact heat evoked potential, LEP: laser evoked potential, ALS: amytrophic lateral sclerosis

In multicentre studies, abnormal sensory NCS were demonstrated in 17-23% of ALS patients using conventional NCS (i.e., median and sural NCS) (Pugdahl et al., 2007 and 2008).

And, pathological studies in patients with ALS also verified involvement in 70–90% of the myelinated sensory fibres (Heads et al., 1991; Hammad et al., 2007; Luigetti et al., 2012). Comparative evaluation of sural biopsies demonstrated severe involvement of myelinated sensory fibres predominating the largest ones (di Trapani et al., 1987). In addition to loss of A-beta afferents, biopsy findings mostly demonstrated several findings like clustered mitochondria, enlarged small vesicles, and neurofilament accumulation (Dyck et al., 1975; Di Trapani et al., 1987; Heads et al., 1991).

Despite these evidences, the commonly accepted statement "sensory nerves are spared in ALS" dominated the perspectives of neurologists and clinical neurophysiologists for years, most probably based on the ALS studies that used conventional NCS.

Relatively late studies reported abnormal NCS (including distal nerves in addition to conventional NCS), SEP, and sural biopsy findings in 72.2%, 56.6%, and 12.2% of advanced stage ALS patients, respectively (Isak et al., 2016 and 2017). Lower extremities were shown to be affected more than upper extremities, and distal NCS were more sensitive than conventional NCS to define the involvement of A-beta fibres. These two observations suggested that the involvement of A-beta fibres were actually more widespread than the previous studies that used conventional NCS. The higher percentages for abnormal neurophysiological tests than abnormal sural biopsies could be referred to alterations in excitabilities in A-beta fibres in addition to neurodegeneration in ALS (Kanai et al., 2006; Nakata et al., 2006; Vucic et al., 2006). Also, the sural biopsies were taken from the ankle potentially could have bypassed the more severely affected distal sections i.e., dorsal sural nerve.

A-Delta Fibres

In ALS, A-delta sensory fibres- elements of nociceptive system, are usually assessed for investigations but not diagnostic purpose (Table 2).

As NCS cannot assess denervation or dysfunction in A-delta or C-fibres, specialized procedures, for example cortical potentials evoked by laser (LEP) or contact heat (CHEP), are used to identify denervation in these fibres (Cruccu et al., 2008; Chen et al., 2001). However, the studies with LEP or CHEP in ALS patients reported conflicting results with each other; e.g., a LEP study suggested affected A-delta fibres in ALS based on increased LEP amplitudes and prolonged LEP latencies (Simone et al., 2010) but the CHEP study suggested spared A-delta fibres (Xu et al., 2009). Both studies had some methodological problems. Firstly, lower extremities were not evaluated in these studies. So, the denervation of A-delta fibres in lower extremities was totally ignored. In additon, the evidences coming from relatively early pathological studies were not fully taken into consideration. Increased LEP amplitudes were explained with compensatory facilitation of the nociceptive cortex and prolonged LEP latencies with affected spinothalamic tract in cortical and subcortical levels (Simone et al., 2010). The first statement is probably true for that patient group but a statement on affected A-delta fibres only in the central nervous system could be a bit insufficient explanation. Pathological evidences in ALS patients confirmed that A-delta fibres were affected not only in the central (Lowe and Leigh 2002) but also in the peripheral nociceptive fibres (Hammad et al., 2007). And, CHEP study seems to have a relatively subjective perspective because the patients with significant sensory abnormalities were excluded (Table 2).

In another study on ALS, A-delta fibres were demonstrated to be affected in 72.2% of the patients using LEPs (Isak et al., 2016). LEPs in lower extremities were more severely affected than upper extremities. Related to disease severity, the LEP results suggested that A-delta fibres were mildly involved in a relatively wide spectrum (Table 2).

C-Fibres

Despite many convincing studies, the involvement of C-fibres in ALS was frequently ignored. The possible reason could be the domination of the clinical picture by weakness and the functional consequences of ALS leading to death.

Stereological and neurophysiological studies showed that the autonomic afferents from visceral organs, skin, and cardiovascular system are composed of myelinated and/or unmyelinated fibres (Duda and Pavlásek, 1975; Fagius and Wallin, 1980; O'Leary and Jones, 2003). But, preganglionic efferents are mainly composed of myelinated fibres (Morgan, 2000). Yet, all the postganglionic fibres are in C-fibre range and are the major determinants of autonomic responses. Therefore, the studies that evaluated autonomic system impairment were presented under C-fibres section (Table 3).

Table 3. Studies that used autonomic tests, corneal confocal microscopy, and laryngeal endoscopy

Author, Issue Year	Tests	Major Results
Shimizu et al., 1992	SRC in peripheral blood vessels following NE injection in respiratory dependent ALS patients	High plasma NE in ALS patients. SRC of ALS patients were similar to controls. Three ALS patients showed hyposensitivity of alpha-adrenal receptors.
Oey et al., 2002	MSNA, BP, HR following valsalva manoeuvre, SSR, ECG and respiration	No orthostatic intolerance in ALS patients. Increased HR decreased BP at rest, reduced MSNA, prolonged SSR latencies in ALS patients. No plantar SSR in 19% of ALS patients.
Pavlovic et al., 2010	Cardiac autonomic tests (power spectrum analysis	Increased power spectrum analysis of RR variability and decreased tine domain parameters of HRV in ALS patients.
Shindo et al., 2011	SSR, Skin blood flow, SSNA	Increased resting SSNA frequency, prolonged SSNA reflex latencies, frequent spontaneous resting SSRs in ALS patients.
Nygren and Fagius., 2011	MSNA and sympatho-excitatory manoeuvres following glucose intake	Reduced glucose tolerance, increased HR, and increased MSNA at rest,, and weak MSNA response to manoeuvres in ALS patients.
Pinto et al.,2012	Autonomic tests in consecutive visits	Maximal, minimal and median HR remained stable in ALS patients. HR coefficient of variation decreased significantly in third visit and three ALS patients died suddenly within two months despite normal pulse oximetry.
Piccione et al., 2015	CASS	Autonomic symptoms in 29% and increased CASS scores in 75% of ALS patients.
Shindo et al., 2015	MSNA, HR, BP, PaO2, PaCO2, and VC%	MSNA, PaO2, PaCO2, or VC% was not correlated with disability in ALS patients.
Shindo et al., 2016	MSNA, HR, and BP	Increased MSNA, and relatively small alterations in HR, BP and frequency of MSNA bursts in head up tilt tests of ALS patients.
Ferrari et al., 2014	Corneal confocal microscopy	Increased tortuosity, and reduced fibre length and corneal fibre density of ALS patients.
Ruoppolo et al., 2016	Endoscopic evaluation of larynx and larynx Bx	49% and 33.3% of the patients had dysphagia and laryngeal sensory deficit, respectively. Abnormal larynx biopsies in three patients

SRC: stimulus response curve, NE: norepinephrine, MSNA: muscle sympathetic nerve activity recorded with microneurography, BP: blood pressure, HR: heart rate, SSR: sympathetic skin response, ECG: electrocardiogram, HRV: heart rate variability, SSNA: skin sympathetic nerve activity, CASS: composite autonomic symptom score, ALS: amyotrophic lateral sclerosis, PAO2: partial oxygen pressure, PaCO2: partial carbon dioxide pressure, VC%: percentage of vital capacity, Bx: biopsy, QST: quantitative sensory testing,

Mild autonomic impairment was demonstrated particularly in the advanced phases of ALS (Shimizu et al., 1995; Oey et al., 2002; Pavlovic et al., 2010; Shindo et al., 2011, 2015 and 2016; Nygren and Fagius, 2011; Pinto et al., 2012; Piccione et al., 2015). Despite the different autonomic protocols used, these studies showed abnormal findings (e.g., abnormally increased heart rates and/or decreased baroreflex sensitivities at rest, reduced muscle or skin sympathetic nerve activities to stress using microneurography, and abnormally prolonged or absent sympathetic skin responses) in ALS patients (Table 3). Many investigators suggest an imbalance predominated by sympathetic over activity and parasympathetic dysfunction during the ALS progression. Supporting this point of view, sudden death due to reduced heart rate variability was presented in some ALS patients (Pinto et al., 2012).

About C-fibres in nociseptive system; most of the studies assessed C-fibre denervation in ALS via skin or nerve biopsies (Heads et al., 1991; Hammad et al., 2007; Luigetti et al., 2012; Devigli et al., 2011; Weis et al., 2011; Truini et al., 2015) (Table 4). One of them was a sural biopsy study and the number of degenerated C-fibres was not different from the controls (Hammad et al., 2007). And, C-fibres were relatively unaffected when compared to degenerations in A-beta and A-delta fibres (73% and 23%, respectively) (Hammad et al., 2007). Another study used skin biopsies and found 79% reduction in intraepidermal nerve fibre density (IENFD), using a cut-off value of 8 fibre/mm (Weis et al., 2011). The reason for choosing 8 fibre/mm cut-off was not explained but the percentage of involvement for C-fibres could have been lower if a quantification based on the normative ranges given by the European Federation of the Neurological Societies was used (Lauria et al., 2010a 2010b). And, a later study compared skin biopsies and thermal detection thresholds of bulbar and spinal onset ALS patients (Truini et al., 2015). The authors reported a reduction of 85% and 9% in IENFDs of spinal and bulbar onset ALS patients, respectively.

Table 4. Studies that used functional (quantitative sensory testing) and structural (nerve or skin biopsies) evaluations

Author, Issue Year	Tests	Major Results
di Trapani et al., 1987	Sural Bx, NCS	Marked loss of myelinated fibres; all types of fibre types are affected predominating in the largest ones.
Heads et al., 1991	Sural Bx	Axonal degeneration, increased re-myelination, and left shift in diameter in sensory fibres of ALS patients.
Hammad el al., 2007	Sural Bx, NCS	Sensory signs and symptoms in 32%, and abnormal sural amp in 27% of ALS patients. Axonal degeneration and regeneration in 91% of ALS patients' biopsies.
Devigli et al., 2011	Sural Bx	Inflammatory cell infiltrates in 61% of ALS patients.
Weis et al., 2011	Skin Bx	Mild sensory symptoms in 25%, C-fibre loss in 79%, and axonal swellings in 60% of ALS patients.
Luigetti et al., 2012	Sural Bx	Axonal loss in 71%, regenerating clusters in 53%, and wallerian degenerations in 35% of ALS patients.
Truini et al., 2015	Sural NCS, thermal QST and skin Bx	Normal sural SNAP in 96% of ALS patients. Abnormal QST and skin Bx findings in 84.6% of spinal-onset and 9% of bulbar onset ALS patients.
Mulder et al., 1983	QST	Increased VT but no change in touch-pressure or thermal cooling thresholds.
Jamal et al., 1985	Thermal QST	Abnormal thermal QST in 80% of the patients.
Deepika et al., 2006	QST	No abnormalities in ALS patients.
Theys et al., 1999	QST, NCS, SEP	At least one abnormal test in 60% of patients. Sural amplitudes were decreased, heating thresholds were elevated, but cooling thresholds were normal in ALS patients.
Isak et al., 2017	QST, Skin Bx, Sural Bx	Abnormal QST, skin Bx, and sural Bx in 12.5%, 9.7%, and 12.5% of ALS patients, respectively.

Bx: biopsy, NCS: nerve conduction studies, QST: quantitative sensory testing, SEP: somatosensory evoked potential, ALS: amyotrophic lateral sclerosis

Another study on skin biopsies in ALS patients evaluated C fibres in epidermis (Isak et al., 2017). The investigators used PGP 9.5 staining to determine IENFD, growth associated protein 43 (GAP 43) staining to determine re-innervation, and axonal swelling ratios (Hsieh et al., 2000;

Lauria et al., 2003; Brown et al., 2000; Cheng et al., 2013). Despite insignificant changes in mean IENFD values of ALS patients and healthy subjects, mild reductions in IENFD were shown in few patients. GAP 43 antibody staining was negative but axonal swelling ratios were increased in C-fibres of all patients. Relatively preserved C fibres in ALS patients could be explained either by a re-innervation process or a relative resistance to neurodegeneration. At this point; negative GAP 43 antibody staining probably pointed out lack of a re-innervation process. Yet, another re-innervation mechanism following a different pathway could still be possible. Therefore, relatively preserved IENFD suggested a relative resistance to neurodegenerative process in C fibres of ALS patients. But, the meaning of axonal swellings was not fully clarified. Axonal swellings can be precursors of C fibre degeneration or re-innervation, or pain generators (Lauria et al., 2010; Cheng et al., 2013; Karlsson et al., 2013 and 2015; Bursova et al., 2012; Scheyyt et al., 2015). Re-innervation hypothesis was not supported because none of the ALS patients had a positive staining for GAP 43 antibody in the skin biopsy material (Isak et al., 2017). Also, the other hypothesis, i.e., axonal swellings on C-fibres could be pain generators, seems unlikely for ALS patients because none of the ALS patients were defined to have neuropathic pain (Isak et al., 2016b). Simply, axonal swellings could be a reflection of dysfunctional axonal transport in ALS similar to axonal spheroids in motor nerves (Hoffman and Griffin, 1993).

In 2018, another potential use of skin biopsy was suggested. In addition to reduced IENFD, sweat gland nerve fibre density, Meissner's corpuscle density, and pilomotor nerve fibre density in skin biopsies, the investigators reported pTDP-43 deposition in nerve fibres of ALS patients as a new potential biomarker to diagnose ALS (Ren et al., 2018).

Alternatively, few studies quantified C-fibres in different organs of ALS patients. One study used corneal confocal microscopy, a technique that enables non-invasive quantitative evaluation of corneal C- nerve fibre density (CNFD), revealed significant reductions in CNFD and corneal nerves total length, and increase in the corneal nerves mean tortuosity (Ferrari et al., 2014). Based on these observations, the authors suggested a subclinical C-fibre involvement in ALS patients. Another study evaluated sensory fibres in larynx of ALS patients via endoscopic evaluation of swallowing and larynx biopsies (Ruoppolo et al., 2016). One third of the patients had laryngeal sensory deficit and larynx biopsies obtained from three patients showed absent IENF in one patient, and abnormal morphological changes in two patients despite normal IENFD.

FUNCTIONAL EVALUATION OF SENSORY INVOLVEMENT

Usually, sensual signs are neither the core complaints in an ALS patient nor the major problem of the physician to investigate (Inghilleri and Iavocelli, 2011). In ALS, symptoms referred to sensory involvement were described in less than one third of the patients (Gubbay et al., 1985; Hammad et al., 2007). Functional evaluation of sensory network (i.e., neurological examinations, QSTs and pain questionnaires) in ALS patients was handled separately because of the discrepancy between the results of neurophysiological tests and functional evaluations (Table 4) (Theys et al., 1999; Mulder et al., 1983; Deepika et al., 2006; Jamal et al., 1985).

Several reasons could be suggested for relatively unnoticed sensory signs and symptoms; Firstly, in ALS, sensory neurons are accepted to be affected less than motor neurons (Hammad et al., 2007). Also weakness could be more disabling than hypoesthesia for the ALS patient and sensory abnormalities in ALS patients are usually sub-clinical (Theys et al., 1999). And, during relatively fast progression of ALS, sensory disturbances in ALS patients could be explained by the nerve compression following supportive braces, immobility, or cachectic state.

Few quantitative sensory testing (QST) studies revealed conflicting results in ALS patients. One study showed normal QST endorsing the statement of intact sensory fibres in ALS (Deepika et al., 2006), while others showed abnormal detection thresholds (Theys et al. 1999; Mulder et al., 1983; Jamal et al., 1985). And, relative vulnerability of thicker sensory fibres than thin fibres in MND was mentioned based on more abnormal results in vibration thresholds (A-beta function) than thermal cooling thresholds (A-delta and C- fibre functions) in ALS patients (Mulder et al., 1983). In anothert study, concordant with skin biopsy results, abnormal thermal detection thresholds were reported in 84% and 9% of the spinal- and bulbar-onset ALS patients, respectively (Truini et al., 2015).

Also, pain was studied as a disabling symptom in ALS patients (Rivera et al., 2013). Pain in ALS patients is primarily attributed to musculoskeletal basis (Borasio et al., 2001). Since sensory fibres are relatively spared in ALS, neuropathic pain is frequently not accepted as the underlying mechanism of pain. However, taking the evidences of sensory involvement into account, the pain due to neuropathic origin could still be suspected in ALS.

In several reports conducted on the same patient group, neurological examinations, a pain questionnaire, and QSTs revealed abnormal findings in 38.8%, 9.7%, and 12.5% of ALS patients, respectively (Isak et al., 2016a, 2016b, and 2017). In neurological examinations of ALS patients, loss of sensory function (i.e., hypoesthesia) was detected but none of the patients reported increased sensory perception (e.g., hyperesthesia or allodynia). Correspondingly, none of the patients had any complaint suggesting neuropathic pain. The authors suggested that, unlike the inflammatory processes (Campbell and Meyer, 2006), sensitization cascades starting from peripheral nociceptors (i.e., peripheral sensitization) followed by central sensitization of spinal and cortical neurons are not triggered in ALS. So, loss of function (e.g., hypoesthesia, anaesthesia) could be expected to be experienced more than gain of function (e.g., hyperesthesia, allodynia) or neuropathic pain in ALS patients.

PATTERN OF SENSORY INVOLVEMENT IN ALS

Many studies investigated sensory involvement in ALS in a limited perspective, i.e., mostly confined to one fibre type using few neurophysiological, functional, or structural parameters. Only a small number of studies tried to look at the big picture to understand the range and pattern of sensory involvement.

A study used NCS, QST, and skin biopsies to compare spinal- and bulbar- onset ALS patients (Truini et al., 2015). Taking percentage of motor neuron involvement 100%; only 4.1% showed abnormal sural NCS, but 85% of the spinal onset and 9% of the bulbar onset patients had abnormal QST and skin biopsy findings (Truini et al., 2015). Their results suggested a pattern similar to diabetic polyneuropathies, i.e., small calibre sensory fibres were affected more than large calibre nerve fibres. On the other hand, an early study used only sural biopsy as the comparative test (Hammad et al., 2007). Again, taking the percentage of motor neuron involvement in ALS patients as 100% into account; abnormal findings were defined in 73% and 23% of A-beta and A-delta sensory fibres, respectively. And, the changes in C- fibres were not different from the controls. These findings suggested a different pattern, i.e., large fibres are affected more than smaller ones. In another study, the same pattern of involvement was reported in ALS patients based on abnormal NCS, LEP, SEP, nerve biopsy, skin biopsy, neurological examination, and QST findings in 72.2%, 72.2%, 56.6%, 12.5%, 9.7%, 38.8%, and 12.5%, respectively (Isak et al.,2016a, 2016b, and 2017). Higher abnormalities in neurophysiological procedures (i.e., NCS, SEP, or LEP) than functional measures (i.e., neurological examination or QST) was explained by the differences in the focus of the diagnostic procedures. NCS, LEP, or SEP reflects the functions (i.e., velocities, latencies, or amplitudes) of the relatively fast and big units within each fibre group. On the other hand, neurological examinations and QST reflect the functions of the minimum number of the relatively slow and small units needed to percept a specific stimulus (e.g., thermal detection thresholds) or the pain induced by the stimulus (e.g., thermal pain thresholds). Reduced sensation in neurological examination reflects a smaller amount of perception than normal with the same stimulus, and increased thresholds in QSTs reflect more than normal number of smallest units to percept a specific stimulus. In a pathological process affecting big units more than the smaller ones (e.g., ALS), the tests evaluating big units could be expected to deteriorate more than the functional measures evaluating the small units within each fibre group.

INVOLVEMENT OF SENSORY PATHWAY IN CENTRAL NERVOUS SYSTEM OF ALS PATIENTS

A proportional decrease in quantity of nerve cells in primary motor and primary sensory cortexes suggesting an interactive degeneration was previously suggested in sporadic ALS patients (Mochizuki et al., 2011). Later, involvement of sensory cortex was demonstrated using volumetric, diffusion tensor imaging(DTI), and functional magnetic resonance imaging (MRI) studies in brain (Meadowcroft et al., 2015, Devine et al., 2015, Thorns et al., 2013, Mohammadi et al., 2011, Konrad et al., 2002, Lule et al., 2010). In addition, degeneration of sensory pathways was demonstrated in spinal cord (Iglesias et al., 2015) (Table 5).

Table 5. Studies that used functional (quantitative sensory testing) and structural (nerve or skin biopsies) evaluations

Author, Issue Year	Tests	Major Results
Meadowcroft et al., 2015	Post mortem MRI and histological assessment	Reduction in cortical grey and subcortical white matters of somatosensory and primary visual networks.
Devine et al., 2015	Brain MRI	Asymmetric grey matter reduction of the left somatosensory cortex and the temporal gyri in right limb onset ALS
Iglesias et al., 2015	Spinal diffusion tensor imaging (DTI) and SEP	Abnormal SEP and DTI of ascending sensory fibres in almost 40% and 60% of patients, respectively.
Mohammadi et al., 2011	Functional MRI	Activations in contralateral somatosensory cortex
Konrad et al., 2002	Functional MRI	Activation in parietal somatosensory cortex

MRI: magnetic resonance imaging, DTI: diffusion tractography imaging, SEP: somatosensory evoked potential, ALS: amyotrophic lateral sclerosis

Involvement of Sensory Fibres in Familial ALS and Other Motor Neuron Diseases

Sensory involvement was described in some patients with famillial ALS, mostly in SOD1 and TARDBP mutations (Camdessanche et al., 2011).

Also, PLS patients, a rare MND affecting mainly upper motor neurons, usually do not complain sensory deficits but abnormal SEPs were reported (Kupiers-Upmajer et al., 2001).

Also, sensory abnormalities were mentioned in other motor neuron diseases (e.g., Kennedy's MND, Hirayama's disease) confined to lower motor neurons (Hama et al., 2012; Polo et al., 2003).

Longer life span in these diseases than ALS could probably make the sensory changes in these diseases relatively apparent in long term.

PRACTICAL SUGGESTIONS AND FUTURE PERSPECTIVES

Taking many supportive studies into consideration, it could be claimed that ALS diagnosis should not be declined based on the findings pointing out sensory denervation. Consequently, sensory findings in neurological examination or neurophysiological procedures should not lead the neurologists or clinical neurophysiologists to exclude ALS, sharply. Future studies with large study groups and repeated tests during the progress of the disease could be designed to understand the deterioration of sensory fibres in the long term. In addition, demonstration of pTDP-43 in peripheral sensory structures e.g., skin biopsy could be considered to verify ALS in suspicious patients who do not fulfil the diagnostic criteria.

REFERENCES

Belsh J. M., Schiffman P. L. 1990. Misdiagnosis in patients with amyotrophic lateral sclerosis. *Arch Intern Med*; 150:2301–5. PMID: 2241438.

Belsh, J. M., Schiffman, P. L. 1996. The ALS patient perspective on misdiagnosis and its repercussions. *J Neurol Sci*; 139(suppl):110–6. doi: 10.1016/0022-510x(96)00088-3.

Borasio, G. D., Voltz, R., Miller, R. G. 2001. Palliative care in amyotrophic lateral sclerosis. *Neurol Clin.*; 19: 829–47. doi: 10.1016/ s0733-8619(05)70049-9.

Bosch, E Pe., Yamada, T., Kimura, J. 1985. Somatosensory evoked potentials in motor neuron disease. *Muscle Nerve*; 8:556 – 62. doi: 10.1002/mus.880080703.

Braak, H., Brettschneider, J., Ludolph, A. C., Lee, V. M., Trojanowski, J. Q., Del Tredici, K. 2013. Amyotrophic lateral sclerosis-a model of corticofugal axonal spread. *Nat Rev Neurol.*; 12:708-14. doi: 10.1038/nrneurol.2013.221.

Brettschneider, J., Arai, K., Del Tredici, K., Toledo, J. B., Robinson, J .L., Lee, E. B., Kuwabara, S., Shibuya, K., Irwin, D. J., Fang, L., Van Deerlin, V. M., Elman, L., McCluskey, L., Ludolph, A. C, Lee, V. M. Y., Braak, H., Trojanowski, J. Q. 2014. TDP-43 pathology and neuronal loss in amyotrophic lateral sclerosis spinal cord. Acta Neuropathol.; 128, 423–37. doi: 10.1007/s00401-014-1299-6.

Brooks, B. R., Miller, R. G., Swash, M., Munsat, T. L., World Federation of Neurology Research Group on Motor Neuron Diseases. 2000. El Escorial revisited: revised criteria for the diagnosis of amyotrophic lateral sclerosis. Amyotroph Lateral Scler Other Motor Neuron Disord. 1:293–9. doi: 10.1080/146608200300079536.

Brown, A. 2000. Slow axonal transport: stop and go traffic in the axon. Nat Rev Mol Cell Biol;1(2):153-6. doi: 10.1038/35040102.

Bursova, S., Dubovy, P., Vlckova-Moravcova, E., Nemec, M., Klusakova, I., Belobradkova, J, Bednarik, J. 2012. Expression of growth-associated protein 43 in the skin nerve fibers of patients with type 2 diabetes mellitus. *J Neurol Sci.*; 315:60–3. doi: 10.1016/j.jns.2011. 11.038.

Camdessanche, Jean-Philippe, Belzil, V. V., Jousserand, G. Rouleau, G. A., Créac'h, C., Convers, P., Antoine, J. C. 2011. Sensory and motor neuronopathy in a patient with the A382P TDP-43 mutation. Orphanet *J. Rare Dis.*; 6: 1172-6-4. doi: 10.1186/1750-1172-6-4.

Campbell, J. N., Meyer, R. A. 2006. Mechanisms of neuropathic pain. Review. Neuron.; 5; 52: 77–92. doi: 10.1016/j.neuron.2006.09.021.

Chen, A. C., Niddam, D. M., Arendt-Nielsen, L. 2001. Contact heat evoked potentials as a valid means to study nociceptive pathways in human subjects. *Neurosci Lett*.; 316:79–82. doi: 10.1016/s0304-3940(01)02374-6.

Cheng, H. T., Dauch, J. R., Porzio, M. T., Yanik, B. M., Hsieh, W., Smith, A G., Singleton, J. R., Feldman, E. L. 2013. Increased axonal regeneration and swellings in intraepidermal nerve fibers characterize painful phenotypes of diabetic neuropathy. *J Pain*; 14:941–7. doi: 10.1016/j.jpain.2013.03.005.

Cornblath, D. R., Kuncl, R. W., Mellits, E. D., Quaskey, S. A., Clawson, L., Pestronk, A., Drachman, D. B. 1992. Nerve conduction studies in amyotrophic lateral sclerosis. *Muscle Nerve*.; 15:1111-5. doi: 10.1002/mus.880151009.

Cosi, V., Poloni, M., Mazzini, L., Callieco, R. 1984. Somatosensory evoked potentials in amyotrophic lateral sclerosis. *J Neurol Neurosurg Psychiatry*; 47:857– 61. doi: 10.1136/jnnp.47.8.857.

Cruccu, G., Aminoff, M. J., Curio, G., Guerit, J. M., Kakigi, R., Mauguiere, F., Rossini, P. M., Treede, R. D., Garcia-Larrea, L. 2008. Recommendations for the clinical use of somatosensory-evoked potentials. Clin Neurophysiol.; 119:1705–19. doi: 10.1016/j.clinph. 2008.03.016.

Dasheiff, R. M., Drake, M. E., Brendle, A., Erwin, C.W. 1985. Abnormal somatosensory evoked potentials in amyotrophic lateral sclerosis. *Electroencephalogr Clin Neurophysiol*.; 60:306-11. doi: 10.1016/ 0013-4694(85)90004-5.

Davenport, R. J., Swingler, R. J., Chancellor, A. M., Warlow, C. 1996. Avoiding false positive diagnoses of motor neuron disease: lessons from the Scottish Motor Neuron Disease Register. *J Neurol Neurosurgery Psychiatry*; 60:147–51. doi: 10.1136/jnnp.60.2.147.

de Carvalho, M., Dengler, R., Eisen, A., England, J. D., Kaji, R., Kimura, J., Mills, K., Mitsumoto, H, Nodera, H., Shefner, J., Swash, M. 2008. Electrodiagnostic criteria for diagnosis of ALS. *Clin Neurophysiol*.; 119:497–503. doi: 10.1016/j.clinph.2007.09.143.

Deepika, J, Manvir, B., Sumit, S., Vinay, G., Trilochan, S., Garima, S., Padma, M. V., Madhuri, B. 2006. Quantitative thermal sensory testing in patients with amyotrophic lateral sclerosis using reaction time exclusive method of levels (MLE). *Electromyogr Clin Neurophysiol.*; 46:145-8. PMID: 16918198.

Devigili, G., Uçeyler, N., Beck, M., Reiners, K., Stoll, G., Toyka, K. V., Sommer, C. 2011. Vasculitis-like neuropathy in amyotrophic lateral sclerosis unresponsive to treatment. *Acta Neuropathol.*; 122:343-52. doi: 10.1007/s00401-011-0837-8.

Devine, M. S., Pannek, K., Coulthard, A., Mccombe, P. A., Rose, S. E., Henderson, R. D. 2015. Exposing asymmetric gray matter vulnerability in amyotrophic lateral sclerosis. *NeuroImage Clin.;* 7:782–7. doi: 10.1016/j.nicl.2015.03.006.

di Trapani, G., David, P., La Cara, A., Tonali, P., Laurienzo, P. 1987. Light and ultrastructural studies in sural biopsies of the pseudopolyneuropathic form of ALS. Adv Exp Med Biol.; 209: 111–9. doi: 10.1007/978-1-4684-5302-7_18.

Duda, P., Pavlásek, J. 1975. Functional differentiation of splanchnic A delta fibres in relation to viscerosomatic reflexes. *Physiol Bohemoslov.*; 24:137–45. PMID: 167390.

Dyck, P. J., Stevens, J. C., Mulder, D. W., Espinosa, R. E. 1975. Frequency of nerve fiber degeneration of peripheral motor and sensory neurons in amyotrophic lateral sclerosis. Morphometry of deep and superficial peroneal nerves. *Neurology*: 25, 781–785. doi: 10.1212/ wnl.25.8.781.

Ertekin, C. 1967. Sensory and motor conduction in motor neurone disease. *Acta Neurol Scand*; 43:499–512. doi: 10.1111/j.1600-0404.1967.tb05756.x.

Fagius, J., Wallin, B. G. 1980. Sympathetic reflex latencies and conduction velocities in normal man. *J Neurol Sci.*; 47:433–48. doi: 10.1016/0022-510x(80)90098-2.

Ferrari, G., Grisan, E., Scarpa, F., Fazio, R., Comola, M., Quattrini, A., Comi, G., Rama, P., Riva, N. 2014. Corneal confocal microscopy reveals trigeminal small sensory fiber neuropathy in amyotrophic lateral sclerosis. Front Aging Neurosci.; 16:6:278. doi: 10.3389/fnagi.2014.00278.

Fincham, R. W., Van Allen, M. W. 1964. Sensory nerve conduction in amyotrophic lateral sclerosis. *Neurology*; 14:31–3. doi: 10.1212/wnl.14.1.31.

Gregory, R., Mills, K., Donaghy, M. 1993. Progressive sensory nerve dysfunction in amyotrophic lateral sclerosis: a prospective clinical and neurophysiological study. *J Neurol.*; 240:309-14. doi: 10.1007/bf00838169.

Gubbay, S. S., Kahana, E., Zilber, N., Cooper, G., Pintov, S., Leibowitz, Y. 1985. Amyotrophic lateral sclerosis. A study of its presentation and prognosis. *J. Neurol*; 232, 295–300. doi: 10.1007/bf00313868.

Hama, T., Hirayama, M., Hara, T., Nakamura, T., Atsuta, N., Banno, H., Suzuki, K., Katsuno, M., Tanaka, F., Sobue, G. 2012. Discrimination of spinal and bulbar muscular atrophy from amyotrophic lateral sclerosis using sensory nerve action potentials. Muscle Nerve; 45:169-74. doi: 10.1002/mus.22291.

Hamada, M., Hanajima, R., Terao, Y., Sato, F., Okano, T., Yuasa, K., Furubayashi, T., Okabe, S., Arai, N., Ugawa, Y. 2007. Median nerve somatosensory evoked potentials and their high-frequency oscillations in amyotrophic lateral sclerosis. *Clin Neurophysiol*; 118:877–86. doi: 10.1016/j.clinph.2006.12.001.

Hammad, M., Silva, A., Glass, J., Sladky, J. T., Benatar, M. 2007. Clinical, electrophysiologic, and pathologic evidence for sensory abnormalities in ALS. *Neurology*; 69:2236–42. doi: 10.1212/01.wnl.0000286948.99150.16.

Heads, T., Pollock, M., Robertson, A., Sutherland, W. H., Allpress, S. 1991. Sensory nerve pathology in amyotrophic lateral sclerosis. *Acta Neuropathol* (Berl); 82:316–20. doi: 10.1007/bf00308818.

Hoffman, P. N., Griffin, J. W. 1993. "The control of axonal calibre" In: *Peripheral neuropathy* edited by Dyck PJ. 389–402. Philadelphia: W. B. Saunders.

Hsieh S,-T., Chiang, H. Y., Lin, W. M. 2000. Pathology of nerve terminal degeneration in the skin. *J Neuropathol Exp Neurol*; 59:297–307. doi: 10.1093/jnen/59.4.297.

Iglesias, C., Sangari, S., El Mendili, M. M., Benali, H., Marchand-Pauve, V., Pradat, P. F. 2015. Electrophysiological and spinal imaging evidences for sensory dysfunction in amyotrophic lateral sclerosis. *BMJ Open.*;5(2):e007659. doi: 10.1136/bmjopen-2015-007659.

Inghilleri, M., Iacovelli, E. Clinical neurophysiology in ALS. Review. 2011. *Arch Ital Biol.*; 149: 57–63. doi: 10.4449/aib.v149i1.1264.

Isak, B., Pugdahl, K., Karlsson, P., Tankisi, H., Finnerup, N.B., Furtula,. J., Johnsen, B., Sunde, N., Jakobsen, J., Fuglsang-Frederiksen, A. 2017. Quantitative sensory testing and structural assessment of sensory nerve fibres in amyotrophic lateral sclerosis. *J Neurol* Sci;373:329–34 doi: 10.1016/j.jns.2017.01.005.

Isak, B., Tankisi, H., Johnsen, B., Pugdahl, K., Finnerup, N. B., Fuglsang-Frederiksen, A. 2016. Laser and somatosensory evoked potentials in amyotrophic lateral sclerosis. Clin Neurophysiol.; 127:3322–8. doi: 10.1016/j.clinph.2016.08.008.

Isak, B., Tankisi, H., Johnsen, B., Pugdahl, K., Møller, A. T., Finnerup, N. B., Christensen, P. B., Fuglsang-Frederiksen, A. 2016. Involvement of distal sensory nerves in amyotrophic lateral sclerosis. Muscle Nerve; 54:1086–92 doi: 10.1002/mus.25157.

Jamal, G. A, Weir, A. I., Hansen, S., Ballanatyne, J. P. 1985. Sensory involvement in motor neuron disease: further evidence form automated thermal threshold determination. *J Neurol Neurosurg Psychiatry*; 48:906–10. doi: 10.1136/jnnp.48.9.906.

Jeremy, D I., Dean, A. F., Shaw, C. E., Al-Chalabi, A., Mills, K., Leigh, P. N. 2007. Amyotrophic lateral sclerosis with sensory neuropathy: part of a multisystem disorder? J Neurol Neurosurg Psychiatry.; 78:750-3. doi: 10.1136/jnnp.2006.098798,

Kanai, K., Kuwabara, S., Misawa, S., Tamura, N., Ogawara, K., Nakata, M., Sawai, S., Hattori, T., Bostock, H. 2006. Altered axonal excitability properties in amyotrophic lateral sclerosis: impaired potassium channel function related to disease stage. *Brain*;129: 953–62. doi: 10.1093/brain/awl024.

Karlsson, P, Møller, A. T., Jensen, T. S., Nyengaard, J. R.. 2013. Epidermal nerve fiber length density estimation using global spatial sampling in healthy subjects and neuropathy patients. *J Neuropathol Exp Neurol*; 72:186–93. doi: 10.1097/NEN.0b013e318284e849.

Karlsson, P., Nyengaard, J. R., Polydefkis, M., Jensen, T. S. 2015. Structural and functional assessment of skin nerve fibres in small-fibre pathology. *Eur J Pain*; 19:1059–1070. doi: 10.1002/ejp.645.

Konrad, C., Henningsen, H., Bremer, J., Mock, B., Deppe, M., Buchinger, C., Turski, P., Knecht, S., Brooks, B. 2002. Pattern of cortical reorganization in amyotrophic lateral sclerosis: a functional magnetic resonance imaging study. *Exp Brain Res.*;143:51–56. doi: 10.1007/s00221-001-0981-9.

Kuipers-Upmajer, J., de Jager, A. E., Hew, J. M., Snoek, J. W., van Weerden, T. W. 2001. Primary lateral sclerosis: clinical, neurophysiological, and magnetic resonance findings. *J Neurol Neurosurg Psychiatry*; 71:615-20. doi: 10.1136/jnnp.71.5.615.

Lauri, A. G., Morbin, M., Lombardi, R., Borgna, M., Mazzoleni, G., Sghirlanzoni, A., Pareyson, D. Axonal swellings predict the degeneration of epidermal nerve fibers in painful neuropathies. *Neurology*. 2003;61:631–6. doi: 10.1212/01.wnl.0000070781. 92512.a4.

Lauria, G., Bakkers, M., Schmitz, C., Lombardi, R., Penza, P., Devigili, G., A Gordon, S., Hsieh, S.-T., Mellgren, S. I., Umapathi, T., Ziegler, D., Faber, C. G., Merkies, I. S. J. 2010. Intraepidermal nerve fiber density at the distal leg: a worldwide normative reference study. *J Peripher Nerv Syst.*; 15:202–7. doi: 10.1111/j.1529-8027.2010. 00271.x.

Lauria, G., Hsieh, S. T., Johansson, O., Kennedy, W. R., Leger, J. M., Mellgren, S. I., Nolano, M., Merkies, I. S. J., Polydefkis, M., Smith, A. G., Sommer, C., Valls-Solé, J, European Federation of Neurological Societies; Peripheral Nerve Society. 2010. European Federation of Neurological Societies/ Peripheral Nerve Society Guideline on the use of skin biopsy in the diagnosis of small fibre neuropathy. Report of a joint task force of the European Federation of Neurological Societies and the Peripheral Nerve Society. *Eur J Neurol*; 17:903–12. doi: 10.1111/j.1468-1331.2010.03023.x.

Lowe, JS, Leigh, N. 2002. "Disorders of movement and system degenerations" In: *Greenfield's neuropathology 7th ed*, edited by Graham DI, Lantos PL. 372–83. New York, NY: Oxford University Press.

Luigetti, M., Conte, A. Del Grande, A., Bisogni, G., Romano, A., Sabatelli, M. 2012. Sural nerve pathology in ALS patients: a single-centre experience. *Neuol Sci*.;33:1095-9 doi: 10.1007/s10072-011-0909-5.

Lule, D., Diekmann, V., Muller, H. P, Kassubek, J., Ludolph, A. C., Birbaumer, N. 2010. Neuroimaging of multimodal sensory stimulation in amyotrophic lateral sclerosis. *J Neurol Neurosurg Psychiatry*.; 81:899–906. doi: 10.1136/jnnp.2009.192260.

Mackenzie, I., Bigio, E. H., Ince, PG., Geser, F., Neumann, M., Cairns, N. J., Kwong, L. K., Forman, M. S., Ravits, J., Stewart, H., Eisen, A., McClusky, L., Kretzschmar, H. A., Monoranu, C. M., Highley, J. R., Kirby, J., Siddique, T., Shaw, P. J., Lee, V. M. Y., Trojanowski, J. Q. 2007. Pathological TDP-43 distinguishes sporadic amyotrophic lateral sclerosis from amyotrophic lateral sclerosis with *SOD1* mutations. *Ann Neurol.*; 61:427–34 doi: 10.1002/ana.21147.

Matheson, J. K., Harrington, H. J., Hallett, M. 1986. Abnormalities of multimodality evoked potentials in amyotrophic lateral sclerosis. *Arch Neurol*; 43:338–40. doi: 10.1001/archneur.1986.00520040026013.

Meadowcroft, M. D., Mutic, N. J., Bigler, D. C., Wang, J. L., Simmons, Z., Connor, J. R., Yang, Q. X. 2014. Histological-MRI correlation in the primary motor cortex of patients with amyotrophic lateral sclerosis: MRI and Histological Analysis of the PMC in ALS. *J Magn Reson Imaging.*;41(3):665–75. doi: 10.1002/jmri.24582.

Mochizuki, Y., Mizutani, T., Shimizu, T., Kawata, A. 2011. Proportional neuronal loss between the primary motor and sensory cortex in amyotrophic lateral sclerosis. *Neurosci Lett.*; 503(1):73-75. doi: 10.1016/j.neulet.2011.08.014.

Mohammadi, B., Kollewe, K., Samii, A., Dengler, R., Münte, T. F. 2011. Functional neuroimaging at different disease stages reveals distinct phases of neuroplastic changes in amyotrophic lateral sclerosis. *Hum Brain Mapp.*;32:750–8 doi: 10.1002/hbm.21064.

Mondelli, M., Rossi, A., Passero, S., Guazzi, G. C. 1993. Involvement of peripheral sensory fibers in amyotrophic lateral sclerosis: electrophysiological study of 64 cases. Muscle Nerve.; 16:166-72. doi: 10.1002/mus.880160208.

Morgan, C. W. 2001. Axons of sacral preganglionic neurons in the cat: I. Origin, initial segment, and myelination. *J Neurocytol.*;30: 523–4 doi: 10.1023/a:1015649419346.

Mulder, D. W., Bushek, W., Spring, E., Karnes, J., Dyck, P. J.. 1983. Motor neuron disease (ALS): evaluation of detection thresholds of cutaneous sensation. *Neurology*; 33:1625-7. doi: 10.1212/wnl.33. 12.1625.

Nakano, T., Nakaso, K., Nakashima, K., Ohama, E. 2004. Expression of ubiquitin-binding protein p62 in ubiquitin-immunoreactive intraneuronal inclusions in amyotrophic lateral sclerosis with dementia: analysis of five autopsy cases with broad clinicopathological spectrum. *Acta Neuropathol.* 107:359–64. doi: 10.1007/s00401-004-0821-7.

Nakata, M., Kuwabara, S., Kanai, K., Misawa, S., Tamura, N., Sawai, S., Hattori, T., Bostock, H. 2006. Distal excitability changes in motor axons in amyotrophic lateral sclerosis. *Clin Neurophysiol*; 117:1444–8. doi: 10.1016/j.clinph.2006.04.005.

Nishihira, Y., Tan, C-F., Onodera, O., Toyoshima, Y., Yamada, M., Morita, T., Nishizawa, M., Kakita, A., Takahash, I. H. 2008. Sporadic amyotrophic lateral sclerosis: two pathological patterns shown by analysis of distribution of TDP-43-immunoreactive neuronal and glial cytoplasmic inclusions. *Acta Neuropathol.*; 116:169 -82. doi: 10.1007/s00401-008-0385-z.

Nygren, I., Fagius, J. 2011. High resting level and weak response of baroreflex-governed sympathetic outflow in amyotrophic lateral sclerosis. *Muscle Nerve*; 43:432-40. doi: 10.1002/mus.21894.

O'Leary, D. M., Jones James, F. X. 2003. Discharge patterns of preganglionic neurones with axons in a cardiac vagal branch in the rat. *Exp Physiol.*;88:711–23. doi: 10.1113/eph8802590.

Oey, P. L., Vos, P. E., Wieneke, G. H., Wokke, J. H. J., Blankestijn, P. J., Karemaker, J. M. 2002. Subtle involvement of the sympathetic nervous system in amyotrophic lateral sclerosis. Muscle Nerve.; 25: 402–8. doi: 10.1002/mus.10049.

Ogata, K., Tobimatsu, S, Furuya, H., Kira, J. 2001. Sporadic amyotrophic lateral sclerosis showing abnormal somatosensory evoked potentials: a report of three cases. *Fukuoka Igaku Zasshi*; 92:242–50. PMID: 11494584.

Pavlovic, S., Stevic, Z., Milovanovic, B., Milicic, B., Rakocevic-Stojanovic, V., Lavrnic, D., Apostolski, S. 2010. Impairment of cardiac autonomic control in patients with amyotrophic lateral sclerosis. *Amyotroph Lateral Scler*; 11:272–6. doi: 10.3109/17482960 903390855.

Piccione, E. A., Sletten, D. M., Staff, N. P., Low, P. A. 2015 Autonomic system and amyotrophic lateral sclerosis. *Muscle Nerve*; 5:676–9. doi: 10.1002/mus.24457.

Pinto, S., Pinto, A., de Carvalho, M. 2012. Decreased heart rate variability predicts death in amyotrophic lateral sclerosis. *Muscle Nerve*; 46: 341–5. doi: 10.1002/mus.23313.

Polo, A., Curro' Doss, I. M., Fiaschi, A, Zanette. G. P., Rizzuto, N. 2003. Peripheral and segmental spinal abnormalities of median and ulnar somatosensory evoked potentials in Hirayama's disease. *J Neurol Neurosurg Psychiatry*; 74:627-32. doi: 10.1136/jnnp.74.5.627.

Pugdahl, K., Fuglsang-Frederiksen, A., de Carvalho, M., Johnsen, B., Fawcett, P. R. W., Labarre-Vila, A., Liguori, R., Nix, W., Schofield, I. S. 2007. Generalised sensory system abnormalities in amyotrophic lateral sclerosis: a European multicentre study. *J Neurol Neurosurg Psychiatry*; 78:746–9. doi: 10.1136/jnnp.2006.098533.

Pugdahl, K., Fuglsang-Frederiksen, A., Johnsen, B., de Carvalho, M., Fawcett, P. R. W., Labarre-Vila, A., Liguori, R., Nix, W. A., Schofield, I. S. 2008. A prospective multicentre study on sural nerve action potentials in ALS. *Clin Neurophysiol.*; 119:1106–10. doi: 10.1016/j.clinph.2008.01.010.

Ren, Y., Liu, W., Li, Y., Sun, B., Li, Y., Yang, F., Wang H., Li M., Cui, F. Huang X. 2018. Cutaneous somatic and autonomic nerve TDP-43 deposition in amyotrophic lateral sclerosis. *J Neurol.*;265:1753-1763. doi: 10.1007/s00415-018-8897-5.

Rivera, I., Ajroud-Driss, S., Casey, P., Heller, S., Allen, J., Siddique, T., Sufit, R.. 2013. Prevalence and characteristics of pain in early and late stages of ALS. *Amyotroph Lateral Scler Frontotemporal Degener.*; 14:369–72. doi: 10.3109/21678421.2012.751614.

Ruoppolo, G., Onesti, E., Gori Maria, C. Schettino, I., Frasca, V., Biasotta, A., Giordano, C. Ceccanti, M., Cambieri, C. Greco, A., Buonopane, C. E., Cruccu G. De Vincentiis, M., Inghilleri, M. 2016. Laryngeal Sensitivity in Patients with Amyotrophic Lateral Sclerosis. Front Neurol.; 28:7:212. doi: 10.3389/fneur.2016.00212.

Scheytt, S., Riediger, N. Braunsdorf, S., Sommer, C., Üçeyler, N. 2015. Increased gene expression of growth associated protein-43 in skin of patients with early-stage peripheral neuropathies. *J Neurol Sci.*; 355:131–7. doi: 10.1016/j.jns.2015.05.044.

Schulte-Mattler, W. J., Jakob, M., Zierz S.. 1999. Focal sensory nerve abnormalities in patients with amyotrophic lateral sclerosis. J Neurol Sci.; 15; 162:189-93. doi: 10.1016/s0022-510x(98)00321-9.

Shimizu, T., Hayashi, H., Hayashi, M., Kato, S., Tanabe, H. 1995. Hyposensitivity of peripheral alpha-receptors in respiratory-dependent amyotrophic lateral sclerosis assessed by intravenous norepinephrine infusion. *Clin Auton Res*; 5:165–9. PMID: 7549419.

Shindo, K., Miwa, M., Kobayashi, F., Nagasaka, T, Takiyama, Y. 2016. Muscle sympathetic nerve activity in frontotemporal lobar degeneration is similar to amyotrophic lateral sclerosis. Clin Auton Res.; 26:1-5. doi: 10.1007/s10286-015-0321-y.

Shindo, K., Tsuchiya, M., Ichinose, Y., Onahara, A., Fukumato, M., Koh, K., Takaki, R., Nobuo, Y. Kobayashi, F., Nagasaka, T., Takiyama, Y. 2015. No relation between sympathetic outflow to muscles and respiratory function in amyotrophic lateral sclerosis. J Neurol Sci.; 15; 358:66-71. doi: 10.1016/j.jns.2015.08.017.

Shindo, K., Watanabe, H., Ohta, E., Nagasaka, T., Shiozawa, Z., Takiyama, Y. 2011. Sympathetic sudomotor neural function in amyotrophic lateral sclerosis. Amyotroph Lateral Scler.; 12:39-44. doi: 10.3109/17482968.2010.508529.

Simone, I. L., Tortelli, R., Samarelli, V., D'Errico, E., Sardaro, M., Difruscolo, O., Calabrese, R., De Vito, F. V., Livrea, P., de Tommaso, M. Laser evoked potentials in amyotrophic lateral sclerosis. *J Neurol Sci.* 2010 15; 288: 106–11. doi: 10.1016/j.jns.2009.09.023

Stålberg, E., Sanders, D. B. 1992. "Neurophysiological studies in amyotrophic lateral sclerosis." In: *Handbook of amyotrophic lateral sclerosis*, edited by Smith RA. 209–35. Marcel Decker Inc.

Theys, P. A., Peeters, E., Robberecht, W. 1999. Evolution of motor and sensory deficits in amyotrophic lateral sclerosis estimated by neurophysiological techniques. *J. Neurol.*; 246: 438–42. doi: 10.1007/s004150050379.

Thorns, J., Jansm, A. H., Peschel, T., Grosskreutz, J., Mohammadi, B., Dengler R., Münte T. F. 2013. Extent of cortical involvement in amyotrophic lateral sclerosis-an analysis based on cortical thickness. *BMC Neurol.*;13:148 doi: 10.1186/1471-2377-13-148.

Truini, A., Biasiotta, A., Onesti, E., Di Stefano, G., Ceccanti, M., La Cesa, S., Pepe, A., C Giordano, C., Cruccu, G., Inghilleri, M. 2015. Small-fibre neuropathy related to bulbar and spinal-onset in patients with ALS. *J Neurol.*; 262:1014–8. doi: 10.1007/s00415-015-7672-0.

Weis J., Katona, I., Müller-Newen, G, Sommer, C., Necula, G., Hendrich, C., Ludolph, A. C., Sperfeld A. D. 2011. Small-fiber neuropathy in patients with ALS. *Neurology*; 76:2024–9. doi: 10.1212/WNL.0b013e31821e553a.

Vucic, S., Kiernan, M. C. 2006. Axonal excitability properties in amyotrophic lateral sclerosis. *Clin Neurophysiol*; 117:1458–66. doi: 10.1016/j.clinph.2006.04.016.

Xu, Y. S., Zhang, J, Zheng, J. Y., Zhang, S., Kang, D. X., Fan, D. S. Fully intact contact heat evoked potentials in patients with amyotrophic lateral sclerosis. *Muscle Nerve*. 2009; 39:735–8. doi: 10.1002/mus. 21232.

BIOGRAPHICAL SKETCH

Baris Isak, MD, PhD

Affiliation: Marmara University Hospital Department of Neurology/ Clinical Neurophysiology.

Education: MD, PhD, MSc.

Research and Professional Experience: Professor of Neurology.

Professional Appointments:
- Medical Doctor- Ankara University Medical School(1999)
- Neurology Specialist- Marmara University Hospital Department of Neurology (2005)
- Master of Science (MSc)- Marmara University Hospital Department of Neurology (2009)
- Guest researcher- Azienda Policlinico Umberto I Università di Roma La Sapienza/ Roma-Italia (2011)
- Clinical Assistant- Aarhus Universitet Neurophysiolohisk Afdeling- Aarhus-Denmark(2011-2012)
- Doctor of Philosophy (PhD)- Aarhus Universitet Neurophysiologisk Afdeling- Aarhus-Danmark (2012-2016)
- Associate Professor- Marmara University Hospital Department of Neurology (2012)
- Professor- Marmara University Hospital Department of Neurology (2019).

Honors:

- Fellowship by European Neurological Society- Università di Roma La Sapienza with the project "Hybridization rather than comparison: a study of Cutaneous Silent Period Recordings with Laser Stimulation"(2011)
- Three year full time fellowship by Aarhus University with the project "Electrophysiological and Pathological Evidence of Sensory Changes in Amyotrophic Lateral Sclerosis"
- CONy Best E-Poster Award at the 11th World Congress on Controversies in Neurology in Athens, Greece, 2017 "Sensory Nerve Fibres are involved in Amyotrophic Lateral Sclerosis."

Publications from the Last 3 Years:

IsakB, Pugdahl K, Karlsson P, Tankisi H, Finnerup NB, Furtula J, Johnsen B, Sunde N, Jakobsen J, Fuglsang-Frederiksen A. Quantitative Sensory Testing and Structural Assessment of Sensory Nerve Fibres in Amyotrophic Lateral Sclerosis. J Neurol Sci. 2017 Feb 15;373:329-334.

Kural MA, Karlsson P, Pugdahl K, Isak B, Fuglsang-Frederiksen A, Tankisi H. Diagnostic utility of distal nerve conduction studies and sural near-nerve needle recording in polyneuropathy. *Clin Neurophysiol.* 2017 Sep;128(9):1590-1595

Ventzel L, Madsen CS, Karlsson P, Tankisi H, Isak B, Fuglsang-Frederiksen A, Jensen AB, Jensen AR, Jensen TS, Finnerup NB. Chronic Pain and Neuropathy Following Adjuvant Chemotherapy. Pain Med. 2017 Sep 23. doi: 10.1093/pm/pnx231.

Kenis-Coskun O, Gunes T, Isak B, Yagci I. Kenis-Coskun O, et al. Intrarater and Interrater Reliability of Heckmatt Scoring System in Amyotrophic Lateral Sclerosis. *J Clin Neurophysiol.* 2020 Mar 4. doi: 10.1097/WNP.0000000000000690.

In: Amyotrophic Lateral Sclerosis
Editor: Julie Sørensen

ISBN: 978-1-53618-193-7
© 2020 Nova Science Publishers, Inc.

Chapter 4

NON-INVASIVE VENTILATION IN ALS

Maurizia Lanza, Anna Annunziata and Giuseppe Fiorentino*
Unit of Respiratory Physiopathology, Monaldi Hospital, Naples, Italy

ABSTRACT

The distinctive feature of ALS is its rapid and severe development: the average survival is three years of the onset of the first symptoms and six months after the start of diaphragmatic dysfunction, in the inadequacy of treatment. Respiratory involvement of ALS is the principal cause of death. During the disease time, ALS is characterized by respiratory failure consequent to respiratory muscles dysfunction as well as bulbar muscles which support the upper airways, developing in dyspnoea and impaired sleep, with consequent severe suffering. Respiratory inability progresses gradually and leads to improved CO_2 in the blood; usually, first, at night during sleep; later, during all the day. Hypercapnia produces compromising clinical manifestations such as sleep disruptions, daytime fatigue, cognitive impairment, and depression. Since 1999 with non-invasive ventilation (NIV) has become an essential part of the treatment of ALS that significantly increases survival, quality of life and cognitive performances. From 2006 to the present time, not only has it been

---

* Corresponding Author's Email: Maurizia.lanza85@gmail.ccom.

demonstrated that non-invasive ventilation (NIV) is challenging to adjust in this setting, but also that NIV must be integrated into multidisciplinary control, taking into description improvement of the disease and the patient's living conditions outside of the hospital. The initial NIV settings are simple, but the progression of the disease, ventilator dependence and upper airway involvement sometimes make long-term adjustment of NIV more complicated, with a significant impact on survival. Adjustment of NIV in ALS shows that correction of leaks, management of obstructive apnoea and compliance to the patient's degree of ventilator dependence improve the prognosis. Non-ventilatory factors also impact the efficacy of NIV, and various answers have been reported and must be applied, including cough assist techniques, control of excess salivation and malnutrition. More advanced use of NIV also needs pulmonologists to master the associated end-of-life palliative care, as well as the modalities of interrupting ventilation when it becomes unreasonable. ALS also impairs cough function, appearing in frequent episodes of bronchial congestion and infection. The ALS patient's family plays a principal role in supportive care and everyday management of treatment, including end-of-life palliative care. The impact on the patient's family is devastating, as a consequence of the mixed motor deficit and respiratory failure and the accelerated course of the disease, for which no therapeutic strategy is available.

Keywords: NIV non invasive ventilation, QoL quality of life, SNIP, sniff nasal inspiratory pressure, VC vital capacity

PRESENTATION OF NIV

Mechanical ventilation is an essential step in the life of patients with ALS. It can be an impression feared and traumatic for the patient and his family, with many beliefs that ventilation is related to the tracheostomy and the end of life. Patients should be informed of this method of treatment. Mitsumoto and Rabkin suggested that supporters to explain the therapy to the patient: "Many assistive devices can greatly help breathing, which if left unattended can reduce energy levels and prevent sleep at night. One of these devices is a ventilator. Non-invasive positive pressure includes an easy-to-use mask that fits your face. It should increase energy and provide better sleep. "It could be added that" this reatment also relieves dyspnea while using ventilatory assistance, but probably even when you breathe independently [1].

RESPIRATORY INVOLVEMENT IN ALS

The progressive degeneration of phrenic motoneurons results in diaphragmatic muscle impairment [2, 3]. In the beginning 2000s, the role of diaphragmatic weakness as the principal cause of inadequate sleep and reduced quality of life in ALS patients was validated [4], although this effect was reported in 1979 [5]. Diaphragmatic dysfunction initially alters REM sleep, when accessory respiratory muscles are damaged, and then extends to include every stage of sleep with the consequent progress of the condition. Arnulf et al. described that some cases are capable of using their accessory muscles when REM sleep, as a sequence of an as yet unexplained phenotypic variation [4]. These authors also confirmed a dramatic decrease of survival due to diaphragmatic involvement (217 vs 620 days), providing a piece of primary physiological evidence in support of the use of NIV in ALS, and validating results of earlier analyses [6, 7]. Following these investigations, diaphragmatic involvement of ALS and the compensation granted by NIV have been the subject of diverse publications and significant developments in treatment that will be examined. NIV supports a dramatic decrease in energy expenditure (− 7% of daily resting energy expenditure), as well as 'cortical resting' via limited effects in diaphragmatic muscle impairment. From the first non-controlled studies printed in 1993 [6] to the randomized controlled trial promulgated in 2006 [8], many studies have confirmed that NIV significantly increases survival, quality of life and cognitive performance in ALS notwithstanding disease progress [6, 7, 9]. The survival gain as a sequence of NIV has been calculated to be seven months [8]. Ten years later, with an increase of the quality of NIV and multidisciplinary control, NIV now gives a median improvement in survival of more than 13 months [10]. This improvement is even recognised in patients with bulbar muscle involvement (muscles controlling speech, mastication and swallowing), examined to be poor aspirants for NIV in 2006, with a survival gain of 19 months over those with non-bulbar phenotypes. The progressive development of survival of ALS patients higher the years has been explicitly shown to be due to the initiation of NIV after 2006 [11]. Georges et al. [12] explained that in more than 80% of cases, NIV was started at a grade of daytime hypoventilation including a median PaCO2 of 48 mm Hg. The cut-off estimation for CO2 used to determine hypoventilation in ALS is PCO2 > 45 mm Hg on arterial blood gases while spontaneous breathing, while resting in a seated state for at least 15 min. There is no support at present concerning the best moment of the day to make arterial blood gases (on waking, in the morning or the evening at bedtime) [13]. The utility of nocturnal transcutaneous carbon dioxide (PtcCO2) in ALS has also been newly emphasized [14], but appropriate attention must be paid to the technical problems of PtcCO2 and its security in certain situations (drift and aberrant values). Simultaneous analysis of the pulse oximetry (SpO2) signal provides the detection of significant values. The PtcCO2 cut-off value to move NIV has not been unequivocally determined at the present time, but a 10-mm Hg increase of PtcCO2 above 50 mm Hg for more than 10 min is classically managed to define nocturnal hypoventilation [13]. All guidelines [15] suggest that the suggestion for NIV be based on pulmonary capacity parameters, nocturnal oximetry or even plasma bicarbonate, although specific recommendations are not incongruous. Nocturnal pulse oximetry % time spent < 90%, > 5% or 10%, VC between < 80% and < 50%, SNIP < 40 cm H2O, MIP < 40 cm H2O to < 60 cm, all of those measures at the recommended cut-off values can increase the misgiving of hypoventilation with differing levels of sensitivity. The viewpoint of the characteristics and rapid change of ALS, three-monthly evaluations are needed to discover the appropriate moment to start NIV. But often, three-monthly assessments of PCO2 are not possible due to the painful and invasive nature of arterial blood gases and the cost of percutaneous determinations. More recently, diaphragm ultrasound has been confirmed to detect those at high risk of hypoventilation. Studies have recently validated the value of the ultrasound of the diaphragm, with a good relationship between the thickening section of the diaphragm with the analysis of VC and PaCO2, although no cut-off value has yet been designated as a suspect of hypoventilation [16, 17]. This procedure would be an interesting choice for pre-NIV follow-up, but ultrasound of the diaphragm is infrequently available external of highly specialized centers.

NIV PROLONG SURVIVAL AND IMPROVE QUALITY OF LIFE IN ALS

Survival of ALS patients is increased if NIV is applied for at least 4 consecutive hours when sleep [18]; sleep hypoxia is significantly corrected by an improvement of sleep quality. NIV can relieve signs, avoid hospitalizations, and promote quality of life (QoL) of ALS patients [19]. Bourke and collaborators also observed that quality of life, as measured by a general and a sleep-dependent scale, increased in subjects with NIV [20]. The positive impact on blood-gas parameters, quality of life, and hypercapnia-associated symptoms was recorded convincingly in different succeeding studies. Importantly, while Bourke et al. found increase ment of sleep-related quality of life in all cases, they abandoned to confirm a life-prolonging effect in subjects with pronounced bulbar involvement [20]. Although it is commonly affirmed that NIV therapy is more intricate in bulbar patients due to hypersalivation and other aggravating factors, more recent investigations have revealed that in bulbar patients effectiveness have a prolonged survival as well [21].

CRITERIA FOR INITIATION NIV

All studies printed since 1993 have promoted NIV in patients with daytime or nocturnal hypoventilation [6] but, only some studies have recommended the so-called early ventilation earlier to start of hypoventilation. There is a high risk of hypoventilation and accelerated progression of ALS patient. Three-monthly estimations are needed to discover the relevant time to initiate NIV. However, three-monthly assessments of PCO2 are not feasible due to the painful and invasive nature of arterial blood gases and/or the cost of percutaneous determinations. A recent survey among 186 ALS specialists showed that FVC was the most significant parameter for US practitioners to decide whether NIV was indicated, while European physicians considered the occurrence of orthopnea and dyspnea as most important [12, 22]. The difference in FVC between sitting and supine positions increases is a parameter to estimate. The EFNS guidelines support starting NIV when at least one respiratory clinical sign or one of the subsequent criteria is present: FVC < 80%, SNIP < 40cm H2O, significant nocturnal desaturation, or pCO2 > 45mmHg (morning blood-gas measurements) [15]. The best study at present to detect hypoventilation is the sniff test30with a sensitivity of 97% for a sniff <40 cm H2O [23]. This is much greater than that of vital capacity (VC), which has a sensitivity of only 58% for a value < 50%. More regular measures are obtained with a mask preferably than a mouthpiece, particularly for patients with a bulbar disease [24]. It is essential for identifying sleep apnea in ALS by relevant diagnostic tests. Polysomnography, oximetry, morning blood gases, and SNIP are diagnostic tools that are easy to apply and may point to sleep apnea. Although prospective studies are missing, current data recommends increasing NIV at night in case of sleep apnea and modification of ventilation parameters to limit upper airway obstruction. In asymptomatic ALS subjects with sleep apnea and without NIV, beginning of NIV seems justified, based on existing research [25]. Dorst J et al. report that continuous positive airway pressure should be avoided because respiratory muscles may exhaust during further disease progression. The utility of nocturnal transcutaneous carbon diox is limited to specific conditions (drift and aberrant values). Simultaneous analysis of the pulse oximetry (SpO2) signal provides detection of unusual values. The PtcCO2 cut-off value to propose NIV has not been unequivocally defined at present, but a 10-mm Hg improvement of PtcCO2 above 50 mm Hg for more than 10 min is indicative for hypoventilation [26]. A currently incomplete question regards the importance of NIV before hypoventilation occurs, the 'early' NIV. A large retrospective study [27] and three small group have shown an increase in survival for patients initiating NIV with VC > 80% predicted [28-29], although this effect was not confirmed when sham NIV was applied in the control group. In practice, subjects with only smallest respiratory signs, typically presenting characteristics of motor disability, are unlikely to continue long-term NIV if the treatment is started prior to showing hypoventilation.

HOW SHOULD ALS PATIENTS BE VENTILATED?

Settings

No precise mode of ventilation has been confirmed to be superior. No variation in terms of efficiency has been confirmed among volume assist-control ventilation, in which the patient obtains a predefined volume of gas, and pressure assist-control ventilation, in which partial pressure assistance is the definite feeling of ventilation and the lack of compensation for leaks. The two leading analytical benefits are that it empowers the subject to make air stacking to assist airway clearance and it is able to overcome obstruction to airflow. This is the favoured mode in invasive ventilation. Some highly experienced teams efficiently use this mode for NIV [30], probably with good efficacy for obstructive results (see below). The principal benefits of pressure assist-control ventilation are that it is more comfortable for the subject and, more importantly, it compensates for leaks. Pressure assist-control ventilation is the favoured mode for NIV, even in ventilator-dependent patients. Survival variations in favour of pressure assist-control ventilation have been recognised in large patient cohorts with a follow-up of 10 years (+13 months under pressure-controlled ventilation (10) vs +10 months under volume-controlled ventilation [31]), although other parts including regional and cultural discrepancies probably consider for this finding.

Table 1. Altered parameters indicating NIV needs

Parameter	Alteration
FVC	Change more than 20% respect to precedent value or <80% of predict
paCO2	> 45mmHg
Sniff test	< 40 cmH2O
PtcCO2	> 50 mm Hg for more than 10 min
Polysomnography	Apnoea or hypopnea index > 5/h
Oxymetry	Time spent below 90% > 20%, or 5 minutes continues

Parameters

Several studies so far have examined the impact of different ventilation modes and parameters on blood gases, clinical symptoms, and survival. Ventilation parameters should be useful for the patient to ensure an acceptable quality of life, as well as adequate compliance. At the same time, they should mimic physiological breathing. One study observed no effect of pressure- *versus* volume-controlled ventilation on serviva [31]. Assisted pressure-controlled ventilation is most usually used in clinical application, which forces a controlled breathing, but allows the patient to trigger added breaths at any time. Also, modern ventilation devices support the description of a target tidal volume and automatically accommodate the inspiratory pressure equally within a predefined range. The defined target tidal volume should be chosen according to physiological values which equal 400–600ml in most patients (corresponding to 8ml/kg body weight). Tidal volumes and needed inspiratory pressures usually provide a solid survey about the ventilatory situation of each patient, although ventilation devices may present mistaken data [32]. In contrast to obstructive lung diseases, ALS patients do not regularly require high inspiratory pressures, nor positive end-expiratory pressure (PEEP). The only study examining the effect of PEEP in 25 ALS patients found that a PEEP of 4cm H2O was associated with a worse quality of sleep compared with 0cm H2O [33]. Although evidence is usually low, it can be assumed that PEEP should be avoided when practicable, although it might be necessary in the case of pneumonia or other pulmonary complications. All commercially available masks can be used. Nasal ventilation allows for more uniform humidification, allows communication and induces a lower rate of obstructive apnoea [34]. Ventilation with a single-limb circuit with intended leak needs a mask leak during expiration. It has the advantages of allowing a more extensive option of mask and the use of low-level inspiratory pressure support is usually sufficient when initiating NIV [35]. Semi-controlled pressure modes (automatic modes with back-up frequency) are preferred, being more effective in ALS than automatic modes. Ventilator settings can then be tailored to guarantee sufficient inspiratory assistance to take regular daytime and nighttime PaCO2. Ventilator settings are then continuously set over the first hours and days of ventilation with 3–5 days usually needed to achieve optimal settings. The effectiveness of ventilation should be estimated at 1 month and periodically re-evaluated. A semi-controlled mode with back-up rate is sufficient, even in 24-h-a-day ventilator-dependent patients [36]. The security of ventilation, the presence of alarms and batteries, the dimensions, simplicity (or complexity) and noise are not better, at present, with either pressure assist-control or volume assist- control ventilators. To increase comfort and adherence, it is possible to set various ventilation modes on modern devices, for example, one for the day and one for the night. Sayas Catalan et al. proposed a more detailed analysis of the cause of obstruction by video laryngoscopy during NIV [35]. Lastly, any authors have described the efficacy of a cervical collar or a mandibular advancement device besides.

Monitoring

It is actively promoted adaptation of ventilator settings and monitoring of the quality of NIV. The subject must have able (e.g., a nasal mask change pressure points for different hours a day. Life support ventilators is several types of masks avail- or a nostril mask) to and to allow eating or talking raised. Following the statement of guidelines for NIV quality monitoring based on nocturnal recordings, Atkeson et al. mentioned a high rate of patient/ventilator asynchrony and verified that poor quality of nocturnal NIV is associated with more reduced survival [38]. Leaks are the principal cause of failure of NIV, in more than half of the cases [39] and must be monitored at each follow-up visit. Ventilator software subtracts straightforward verification of leaks, from data card downloads or by tele transmission. Revision of leaks is now relatively simple as a result of the extensive range of masks available on the market [40]. After changing any leaks, the main problem continues obstructive apnoea, which additionally negatively impacts survival when it is not altered.

Ventilation Masks

Evidence concerning the efficacy of various masks for NIV in ALS is absent. The critical issue about which masks should be used has been completely ignored in clinical studies so far. Nasal masks can be doubtful in bulbar patients, because ventilation air might escape due to inadequate closure of the mouth, particularly at night during sleep. On the other hand, nasal masks are usually better tolerated and allow more accessible communication compared with full-face masks covering mouth and nose. Both varieties of the mask can lead to facial pressure ulcers, which may limit their application, and necessitate the use of total full- face masks that cover the whole face but have the disadvantage of more significant dead space and leakage. One study revealed that facial pressure ulcers could- not be prevented by protective patches [41]. In cases with functioning mouth muscles, daytime mouthpiece ventilation may be helpful due to the decreased risk of facial pressure ulcers because even improved speech and swallowing [42].

In summary, there are numerous interfaces, and it is necessary to have many options available to be able to offer the patient the best possible solution. Nevertheless, it is sometimes necessary to use homemade masks for specific patient needs. Frequently, to avoid decubitus, (Figure 1), it is necessary to switch between multiple interfaces during the day and night.

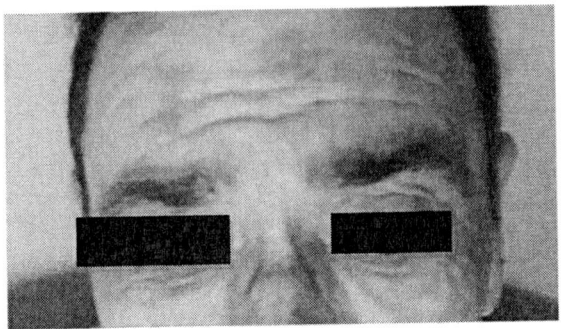

Figure 1. Frontal and nasal decubitus.

MPV and IAPV

Different conditions can also be responsible for the failure of NIV, including claustrophobia, mask-induced skin injuries and rhinitis, with solutions the same as those utilised in other diseases. Other daytime NIV procedures must be considered in highly ventilator-dependent patients in addition to mask ventilation. Mouthpiece ventilation [43] has been recently tested in ALS and can be moved to ventilator-dependent patients who still preserve good orofacial muscle conrecently used in a very preliminary trial in five ALS patients, with attractive sights provided unique also available in a few centres, but has never been studied in ALS. In subjects showing lower NIV tolerance with oronasal and nasal masks, mouthpiece ventilation should always be considered. In patients using NIV many hours a day or in the case of skin lesions, eye irritation, or gastric distention, mouthpiece ventilation should be also contemplated. The use of mouthpiece ventilation combined with other interfaces can lead to an improvement in QoL and greater adherence in ALS patients. Intermittent abdominal compression ventilation (Figure 2) is it consists of a corset with an elastic inflatable bladder that fits over the abdomen. The bladder is attached by a hose to a ventilator that give up to 2.5 liter of air to the bladder and, whereby, to the abdominal wall. This raises the diaphragm to cause expiration below the functional residual capacity. New models avoid clothing taking on the corset buckles and are more comfortable. They are now lightweight, suitable, easy to done and fit and employ velcro for fastening (Figure 2) [44]. But, mouthpiece NVS users generally prefer mouthpiece NVS because of the greater inspiratory volumes that can be taken.

FAILURE OF NIV IN ALS

Congestion due to Excess Salivation

Excess salivation can be a distinct problem of failure of NIV in ALS. Different drugs can be utilised (atropine, scopolamine and belladonna tincture), although salivary gland radiotherapy has been shown to be very useful and should be offered to these patients, even in subjects already treated [45, 46]. Undernutrition is after swallowing dysfunctions and the necessity for gastrostomy. Swallowing disorders, wanting as feeding gastrostomy, can occur after initiating NIV. Various clarifications have been proposed including endoscopic gastrostomy with NIV support [47], but this is difficult to make in patients with severe bulbar lesions who are unable to control mouth leaks during NIV, or percutaneous endoscopic gastrostomy with NIV support which can sometimes be improbable in the presence of very advanced diaphragmatic dysfunction with the intrathoracic stomach. Surgical gastrostomy may sometimes be necessary under brief general anaesthesia with intubation and rapid extubation followed by NIV support [48].

Hypersalivation

Hypersalivation interfere mask ventilation, decreases compliance [31] and worsens prognosis after NIV initiation [49]. Although the pilot study by Bourke and co-workers could not prove a survival benefit of NIV for patients with severe bulbar involvement [8], more current studies oppose this early result. About the diverging results, optimal treatment of NIV limiting symptoms in bulbar patients appears to be a fundamental aspect, and it has been shown that such patients especially benefit from a specialized multidisciplinary setting in hospital [50]. The level of evidence concerning symptomatic therapy of sialorrhea in ALS is usually low. The EFNS guidelines suggest amitriptyline, oral or transdermal hyoscine, or sublingual atropine drops, while the NICE guidelines additionally consider glycopyrrolate, particularly for patients with cognitive impairment, because of fewer central nervous side effects. Injection of botulinum toxin B in the parotid and submandibular glands has been confirmed to increase hypersalivation in about 80% of patients [51] and is regularly applied if patients do not respond adequately to anticholinergic drugs. In our practice, NIV tolerance can be improved considerably in patients with hypersalivation when all available measures are considered. Some authors recommend radiation therapy of salivary glands [45] in patients who do not respond adequately to treatment, but randomized controlled studies are missing.

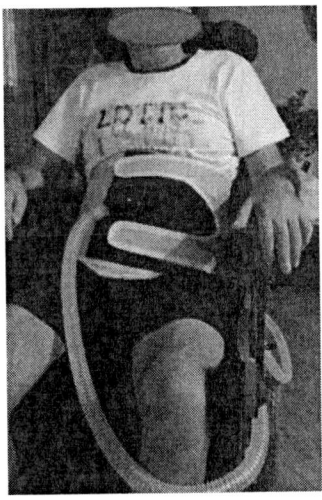

Figure 2. Patient dependent from NIV during IAPV.

Viscous Bronchial Secretions

Thin saliva has to be identified from viscous bronchial secretions that affect patients with disabled coughing and may start to panic attacks and suffocation emotions under NIV. The EFNS and NICE guidelines support nebulizers with saline, anticholinergic bronchodilators, or furosemide [15], as well as humidification of room and ventilation air to decrease or dilute the mucus. Other therapy choices combine mucolytics like N-acetylcysteine and beta-receptor antagonists similar propranolol. Nevertheless, the level of evidence for mucolytic drugs is frequently low, and such agents maybe even serious in patients who cannot effectively expel secretions. Therefore, in our practice, mucolytics should only be practised in sequence with mechanical insufflation–exsufflation (MI-E; 'cough-assist') devices. Such devices have been shown to promote respiratory outcome parameters in ALS [52, 53] while the increase of high-frequency oscillation does not accept any additional advantage [54]. Bulbar patients may not generate sufficient PCF levels under MI-E due to collapse of the upper airways while exsufflation. A randomized controlled study in 40 patients found no differences regarding the frequency of chest infections, quality of life, and survival among MI-E and use of a breath-stacking technique using a lung-volume recruitment bag [55], proposing the latter as a low- cost option. MI-E may be mixed with physiotherapeutic expiration and inspiration manoeuvres, such as manually served cough or air stacking. Some studies have explained that PCF can be raised by these measures [56, 57]. In our practice, cough-assist devices should be used in patients with severe, adhesive secretions in order to free the upper airways before specific ventilation session. This way, it is possible to improve the ventilation comfort and to extend ventilation times. Moreover, in our experience, early education of patients and caregivers regarding airway-clearing techniques has positive effects.

Tracheostomy is Not Systematically the Next Step after NIV

In ALS patients developing acute respiratory failure and intubation, the prognosis is not constantly designated by complete ventilator necessity. It is essential to assess every single case. The opportunity of tracheotomy should be understood by patients with ALS, in any case [58]. On the basis of information level possible today, if the respiratory deficit is severe and NIV is ineffective, the alternative to NIV or death is invasive ventilation. This situation can only be effectively supported by a multidisciplinary team of specialists who contribute decisions collectively with patients and caregivers, regarding the will and dignity of the person. Tracheostomy has been shown to improve survival markedly, as recently highlighted by Stephen Hawking's very long-term survival, with quality of life considered to be adequate by patients [59, 60] although restricted so by caregivers. Any patients and their families although need tracheostomy and they must be implicated as thoroughly as potential about the importance of this decision, ideally as early as practicable, to avoid performing tracheostomy in an acute setting when the subject and the family have not had time to examine this possibility. Mitsumoto and Rabkin [1] have proposed several examples of how tracheostomy can be presented to patients and parents. Development of the quality and efficacy of NIV, even in ventilator-dependent patients, and limited discussions about the provision of ventilation other than with NIV reasonably explain the shallow rate of tracheotomized patients in Western countries. The situation develops to be increasing in Japan [61] where the comparatively automated conversion from NIV to tracheostomy has been decreasing over recent years with patients who have used NIV for more than 6 months being less inclined to request tracheostomy There is no globally accepted guideline regarding implication criteria and the correct time when IV should be granted. Because of its invasiveness and excessive demands of care, it is usually marked as a late choice for sufferers who can no elongated be stabilized by NIV, or who do not tolerate it. But, in circumstances of severe bulbar involvement with massive secretion problems, IV may be estimated earlier. Survival can be prolonged considerably by IV [62], which implies that patients experience far advanced stages of the disease up to develop paralysis and locked-in syndrome. Various subjects refuse IV because they do not feel that quality of life is acceptable under such conditions. It has also been confirmed that subjects who practised NIV for more than 6 months were more inclined to reject tracheostomy [61]. Determination making regarding life-prolonging measures in ALS is a constant process, and patients' choices may change over time. Patients' views toward beginning and end of life-prolonging measures also largely depend on educational setting [63]. In this setting, patients must be informed in particular about the effect of IV at a time when they are informed and the respiratory status is still stationary because it has been shown that family members, as well as inexperienced physicians [64], often underestimate quality of life of ALS subjects and consequently cannot reliably determine his or her own will. A contemporary study revealed that the timing of end-of-life consultations varies greatly [65].

End Life Management

Several symptoms accompanies end of life: dyspnoea, weakness, physical fatigue, reduced support therapy. Symptomatic therapies for dyspnoea so as opioids should be immediately accessible, even relatively early in the development of the disease, if dyspnoea is not adequately mitigated by NIV [15]. A definite association between dyspnoea and pain has been described in subjects who are adequately helped by NIV. According to one study, subjects may undergo psychological weakness and lack of impulse, distress and pain when the last period of life [66]. Physicians experienced in palliative care are regularly able to appropriately maintain the final stage of ALS in an outpatient setting. Nevertheless, the opportunity to be managed at home extensively depends on the availability of sufficient care facilities. When the final phase of the illness, NIV is regularly extended in order to bypass situations of critical dyspnea. Ventilation-dependent subjects who choose to terminate NIV or IV treatment abruptly should ordinarily be diagnosed and managed in a hospital context and should be supported by expert specialists. Diagnostic methods have to include examination and differential analysis of depression that happens alone from physical disability. In cases who do not tolerate ventilation-free intervals, constant profound sedation is required [67]. The patients will need always be asked to plan therapeutic interventions and make decisions on the end or maintenance of life. In the presence of communicated directives, they are taken into statement with the assistance of family members. In the deficiency of advance directives, the patient's will must be ascertained. For this reason, it would be acceptable for the patient to have notice on this, in time to be able to determine how to end life. An approach directive may help to bypass undesired actions. It should be as accurate as practicable and involve the patient's attitude proceeding NIV, IV, and PEG. Patients should be informed about the legal concerns about withdrawal from life-prolonging measures, and support in forming the advance directive should be offered. If end of IV is legal in the patient's country, the progress directive should include whether ventilation should be terminated under specified conditions. Many patients describe the state of complete locked-in syndrome with an inability to drive their eyes as the time to finish life-pro- longing measures [67]. Patients should be informed that death ordinarily occurs peacefully as a result of carbon dioxide narcosis and that fear of suffocation is unfounded, although dyspnea may happen if respiratory complexities like pneumonia occur which may need hospitalization and appropriate therapy. Indicative therapy with opioids, benzodiazepines, and oxygen can sometimes be required to avoid or decrease dyspnea and anxiety. As in some situation of end-of-life dyspnoea, opioids and benzodiazepines, possibly linked with the prescription of oxygen, completely reduce the symptoms caused by discontinuation of ventilatory support. It is only universal sense to begin these procedures before suspending ventilatory support, which can be legitimately instantly continued if the doses administered are inadequate to relieve the patient's symptoms and promote patient comfort. It is essential to ensure the continuous presence of a doctor or a nurse in the patient's room after discontinuing ventilatory support, to allow a rapid answer when the doses need to be increased to reassure the pain thresholds.

CONCLUSION

It has been verified for various years that NIV increases survival and quality of life for patients with ALS and respiratory insufficiency. Contemporary studies have increased the spectrum of subjects who might avail of NIV, including subjects with critical bulbar involvement. Moreover, numerous studies recommend that NIV should be initiated earlier, as recommended by current guidelines, and that NIV can increase survival and respiratory deterioration even in asymptomatic subjects with an FVC > 80%. In this setting, the interrogation, which diagnostics offer the greatest sensibility for discovery of early respiratory insufficiency, is essential. Present studies managing nocturnal capnometry and polygraphy have shown that various patients even with regular FVC undergo from sleep disorders associated to intermittent oxygen desaturations and hypercapnia. In these circumstances, the critical role of sleep apnea in ALS has been frequently identified. These conclusions suggest that respiratory diagnostics should be displayed even in asymptomatic patients, and that NIV should be initiated as promptly as early pathologic variations emerge. Accordingly, randomized controlled studies are required. Original studies have also highlighted the influence of diverse setting circumstances in forms of successfully establishing NIV. Consequently, hypersalivation, as well as viscous bronchial secretions, must be managed to facilitate adequate ventilation. In this context, some recent studies have discussed the corrective choice of MI-E. Although positive experiences are frequently reported, high-level data is still needing. The same concerns to other symptomatic non-invasive treatments of hypersalivation and bronchial secretions in ALS. NIV in patients with neurobehavioral irregularities represents a challenge and should be performed in a specialized, multidisciplinary setting. Although it has been shown that such subjects have a worse agreement and prognosis, current data does not allow the termination that NIV is not indicated in these cases. ALS is a complex disease. Subjects are always heavily addicted on medical care and NIV. Evidence concerning optimal parameter contexts, ventilation masks, and time intervals of NIV usage is still mostly missing, and contemporary practice principally relies on local expertise and experience. The proper timing of the transition from NIV to IV has been neglected by current literature so far. However, the significance of early and extensive patient knowledge about life-prolonging actions and their implications, as well as the presence of a specific multidisciplinary team is generally affirmed.

REFERENCES

[1] Mitsumoto, H; Rabkin, JG. Palliative care for patients with amyotrophic lateral sclerosis: "prepare for the worst and hope for the best". *JAMA*, 2007, 298, 207-216.

[2] Pinto, S; Geraldes, R; Vaz, N; Pinto, A; de Carvalho, M. Changes of the phrenic nerve motor response in amyotrophic lateral sclerosis: longitudinal study. *Clin. Neurophysiol.*, 2009, 120, 2082–5.

[3] Similowski, T; Attali, V; Bensimon, G; Salachas, F; Mehiri, S; Arnulf, I; Lacomblez, L; Zelter, M; Meininger, V; Derenne, JP. Diaphragmatic dysfunction and dyspnoea in amyotrophic lateral sclerosis. *Eur. Respir. J.*, 2000, 15, 332–7.

[4] Arnulf, I; Similowski, T; Salachas, F; Garma, L; Mehiri, S; Attali, V; Behin-Bellhesen, V; Meininger, V; Derenne, JP. Sleep disorders and diaphragmatic function in patients with amyotrophic lateral sclerosis. *Am. J. Respir. Crit. Care Med.*, 2000, 161, 849–56.

[5] Minz, M; Autret, A; Laffont, F; Beillevaire, T; Cathala, HP; Castaigne, P. A study on sleep in amyotrophic lateral sclerosis. *Biomedicine*, 1979, 30, 40–6.

[6] Bach, JR. Amyotrophic lateral sclerosis. Communication status and survival with ventilatory support. *Am. J. Phys. Med. Rehabil.*, 1993, 72, 343–9.

[7] Pinto, AC; Evangelista, T; Carvalho, M; Alves, MA; Sales Luis, ML. Respiratory assistance with a non-invasive ventilator (Bipap) in MND/ALS patients: survival rates in a controlled trial. *J. Neurol. Sci.*, 1995, 129*(Suppl.)*, 19–26.

[8] Bourke, SC; Tomlinson, M; Williams, TL; Bullock, RE; Shaw, PJ; Gibson, GJ. Effects of non-invasive ventilation on survival and quality of life in patients with amyotrophic lateral sclerosis: a randomised controlled trial. *Lancet Neurol.*, 2006, 5, 140–7.

[9] Newsom-Davis, IC; Lyall, RA; Leigh, PN; Moxham, J; Goldstein, LH. The effect of non-invasive positive pressure ventilation (NIPPV) on cognitive function in amyotrophic lateral sclerosis (ALS): a

prospective study. *J. Neurol. Neurosurg. Psychiatry*, 2001, 71, 482–7.

[10] Berlowitz, DJ; Howard, ME; Fiore, JFJ; Vander, Hoorn, S; O'Donoghue, FJ; Westlake, J; Smith, A; Beer, F; Mathers, S; Talman, P. Identifying who will benefit from non-invasive ventilation in amyotrophic lateral sclerosis/motor neurone disease in a clinical cohort. *J. Neurol. Neurosurg. Psychiatry*, 2016, 87, 280–6.

[11] Gordon, PH; Salachas, F; Bruneteau, G; Pradat, PF; Lacomblez, L; Gonzalez-Bermejo, J; Morelot-Panzini, C; Similowski, T; Elbaz, A; Meininger, V. Improving survival in a large French ALS center cohort. *J. Neurol.*, 2012, 259, 1788–92.

[12] Georges, M; Golmard, JL; Llontop, C; Shoukri, A; Salachas, F; Similowski, T; Morelot-Panzini, C; Gonzalez-Bermejo, J. Initiation of non-invasive ventilation in amyotrophic lateral sclerosis and clinical practice guidelines: single-centre, retrospective, descriptive study in a national reference centre. Amyotroph. LateralScler. *Frontotemporal Degener.*, 2017, 18, 46–52.

[13] Piper, AJ; Janssens, JP; Gonzalez-Bermejo, J. Sleep hypoventilation: diagnostic considerations and technological limitations. *Sleep Med. Clin.*, 2014, 9, 301–13.

[14] Kim, SM; Park, KS; Nam, H; Ahn, SW; Kim, S; Sung, JJ; Lee, KW. Capnography for assessing nocturnal hypoventilation and predicting compliance with subsequent noninvasive ventilation in patients with ALS. *PLoS One*, 2011, 6, e17893.

[15] Andersen, PM; Abrahams, S; Borasio, GD; de Carvalho, M; Chio, A; Van Damme, P; Hardiman, O; Kollewe, K; Morrison, KE; Petri, S; et al. EFNS guidelines on the clinical management of amyotrophic lateral sclerosis (MALS) – revised report of an EFNS Task Force. *Eur. J. Neurol.*, 2012, 19, 360–75.

[16] Hiwatani, Y; Sakata, M; Miwa, H. Ultrasonography of the diaphragm in amyotrophic lateral sclerosis: clinical significance in assessment of respiratory functions. Amyotroph. Lateral Scler. *Frontotemporal Degener.*, 2013, 14, 127–31.

[17] Fantini, R; Mandrioli, J; Zona, S; Antenora, F; Iattoni, A; Monelli, M; Fini, N; Tonelli, R; Clini, E; Marchioni, A. Ultrasound assessment of diaphragmatic function in patients with amyotrophic lateral sclerosis. *Respirology*, 2016, 21, 932–8.

[18] Berlowitz, DJ; Howard, ME; Fiore, JF; Jr. et al. Identifying who will benefit from non-invasive ventilation in amyotrophic lateral sclerosis/motor neurone disease in a clinical cohort. *J Neurol Neurosurg Psychiatry.*, Epub ahead of print 11 April 2015. DOI: 10.1136/jnnp-2014-310055.

[19] Radunovic, A; Annane, D; Rafiq, MK; et al. Mechanical ventilation for amyotrophic lateral sclerosis/motor neuron disease. *Cochrane Database Syst Rev*, 2017, 6, CD004427.

[20] Bourke, SC; Tomlinson, M; Williams, TL; et al. Effects of non-invasive ventilation on survival and quality of life in patients with amyotrophic lateral sclerosis: a randomised controlled trial. *Lancet Neurol*, 2006, 5, 140–147.

[21] Bach, JR. Amyotrophic lateral sclerosis: prolongation of life by noninvasive respiratory aids. *Chest.*, 2002, 122(1), 92–98.

[22] Jacobs, TL; Brown, DL; Baek, J; et al. Trial of early noninvasive ventilation for ALS: a pilot placebo-controlled study. *Neurology*, 2016, 87, 1878–1883.

[23] Morgan, RK; McNally, S; Alexander, M; Conroy, R; Hardiman, O; Costello, RW. Use of sniff nasal-inspiratory force to predict survival in amyotrophic lateral sclerosis. *Am. J. Respir. Crit. Care Med.*, 2005, 171, 269–74.

[24] Banerjee, SK; Davies, M; Sharples, L; Smith, I. The role of facemask spirometry in motor neuron disease. *Thorax*, 2013, 68, 385–6.

[25] Heiman-Patterson, TD; Cudkowicz, ME; De Carvalho, M; et al. Understanding the use of NIV in ALS: results of an international ALS specialist survey. *Amyotroph Lateral Scler Frontotemporal Degener*, 2018, 19, 331–341.

[26] Dorst, J; Ludolph, AC. Non-invasive ventilation in amyotrophic lateral sclerosis. *Ther Adv Neurol Disord.*, 2019 Jun 21, 12,

1756286419857040. doi: 10.1177/1756286419857040. PMID: 31258624, PMCID: PMC6589990.

[27] Vitacca, M; Montini, A; Lunetta, C; Banfi, P; Bertella, E; De Mattia, E; Lizio, A; Volpato, E; Lax, A; Morini, R; et al. Impact of an early respiratory care programme with non-invasive ventilation adaptation in patients with amyotrophic lateral sclerosis. *Eur. J. Neurol.*, 2018, 25, 556–e33.

[28] Carratu, P; Spicuzza, L; Cassano, A; Maniscalco, M; Gadaleta, F; Lacedonia, D; Scoditti, C; Boniello, E; Di Maria, G; Resta, O. Early treatment with noninvasive positive pressure ventilation prolongs survival in amyotrophic lateral sclerosis patients with nocturnal respiratory insufficiency. *Orphanet J. Rare Dis.*, 2009, 4, 10.

[29] Jacobs, TL; Brown, DL; Baek, J; Migda, EM; Funckes, T; Gruis, KL. Trial of early noninvasive ventilation for ALS: a pilot placebo-controlled study. *Neurology*, 2016, 87, 1878–83.

[30] Sancho, J; Servera, E; Morelot-Panzini, C; Salachas, F; Similowski, T; Gonzalez-Bermejo, J. Non-invasive ventilation effectiveness and the effect of ventilatory mode on survival in ALS patients. Amyotroph. Lateral Scler. *Frontotemporal Degener.*, 2014, 15, 55–61.

[31] Sancho, J; Martinez, D; Bures, E; Diaz, JL; Ponz, A; Servera, E. Bulbar impairment score and survival of stable amyotrophic lateral sclerosis patients after noninvasive ventilation initiation. *ERJ Open Res.*, 2018, 4, 00159-2017.

[32] Contal, O; Vignaux, L; Combescure, C; et al. Monitoring of noninvasive ventilation by built-in software of home bilevel ventilators: a bench study. *Chest*, 2012, 141, 469–476.

[33] Crescimanno, G; Greco, F; Arrisicato, S; et al. Effects of positive end expiratory pressure administration during non-invasive ventilation in patients affected by amyotrophic lateral sclerosis: a randomized crossover study. *Respirology*, 2016, 21, 1307–1313.

[34] Schellhas, V; Glatz, C; Beecken, I; Okegwo, A; Heidbreder, A; Young, P; Boentert, M. Upper airway obstruction induced by non-

invasive ventilation using an oronasal interface. *Sleep Breath.*, 2018, 22, 781–8.

[35] De Mattia, E; Falcier, E; Lizio, A; Lunetta, C; Sansone, VA; Barbarito, N; Garabelli, B; Iatomasi, M; Roma, E; Rao, F; et al. Passive versus active circuit during invasive mechanical ventilation in subjects with amyotrophic lateral sclerosis. *Respir. Care*, 2018, 63, 1132–8.

[36] Vrijsen, B; Buyse, B; Belge, C; Vanpee, G; Van Damme, P; Testelmans, D. Randomized cross-over trial of ventilator modes during non-invasive ventilation titration in amyotrophic lateral sclerosis. *Respirology*, 2017, 22, 1212–8.

[37] Sayas Catalan, J; Jimenez Huerta, I; Benavides Manas, P; Lujan, M; Lopez-Padilla, D; Arias Arias, E; Hernandez Voth, A; Rabec, C. Video-laryngoscopy with noninvasive ventilation in subjects with upper-airway obstruction. *Respir. Care*, 2017, 62, 222–30.

[38] Atkeson, AD; Roychoudhury, A; Harrington-Moroney, G; Shah, B; Mitsumoto, H; Basner, RC. Patient-ventilator asynchrony with nocturnal noninvasive ventilation in ALS. *Neurology*, 2011, 77, 549–55.

[39] Gonzalez-Bermejo, J; Morelot-Panzini, C; Arnol, N; Meininger, V; Kraoua, S; Salachas, F; Similowski, T. Prognostic value of efficiently correcting nocturnal desaturations after one month of non-invasive ventilation in amyotrophic lateral sclerosis: a retrospective monocentre observational cohort study. *Amyotroph. Lateral Scler. Frontotemporal Degener.*, 2013, 14, 373–9.

[40] Carlucci, A; Schreiber, A; Mattei, A; Malovini, A; Bellinati, J; Ceriana, P; Gregoretti, C. The configuration of bi-level ventilator circuits may affect compensation for non-intentional leaks during volume-targeted ventilation. *Intensive Care Med.*, 2012, 39, 59–65.

[41] Riquelme; MH; Wood; VD; Martinez; FS. Face protective patches do not reduce facial pressure ulcers in a simulated model of non-invasive ventilation. *Rev Chil Pediatr*, 2017, 88, 354–359.

[42] Pinto; T; Chatwin; M; Banfi; P. Mouthpiece ventilation and complementary techniques in patients with neuromuscular disease: a

brief clinical review and update. *Chron Respir Dis*, 2017, 14, 187–193.

[43] Bedard, ME; McKim, DA. Daytime mouthpiece for continuous noninvasive ventilation in individuals with amyotrophic lateral sclerosis. *Respir. Care*, 2016, 61, 1341–8.

[44] Banfi, P; Volpato, E; Bach, JR. Efficacy of new intermittent abdominal pressure ventilator for post-ischemic cervical myelopathy ventilatory insufficiency. *Multi discip Respir Med.*, 2019, 14, 4.

[45] Assouline, A; Levy, A; Abdelnour-Mallet, M; Gonzalez-Bermejo, J; Lenglet, T; Le Forestier, N; Salachas, F; Bruneteau, G; Meininger, V; Delanian, S; et al. Radiation therapy for hypersalivation: a prospective study in 50 amyotrophic lateral sclerosis patients. *Int. J. Radiat. Oncol. Biol. Phys.*, 2014, 88, 589–95.

[46] Amador Mdel, M; Assouline, A; Gonzalez-Bermejo, J; Pradat, PF. Radiotherapy treatment of sialorrhea in patients with amyotrophic lateral sclerosis requiring non-invasive ventilation. *J. Neurol.*, 2015, 262, 1981–3.

[47] Boitano, LJ; Jordan, T; Benditt, JO. Noninvasive ventilation allows gastrostomy tube placement in patients with advanced ALS. *Neurology*, 2001, 56, 413–4.

[48] Gregory, S; Siderowf, A; Golaszewski, AL; McCluskey, L. Gastrostomy insertion in ALS patients with low vital capacity: respiratory support and survival. *Neurology*, 2002, 58, 485–7.

[49] Peysson, S; Vandenberghe, N; Philit, F. Factors predicting survival following noninvasive ventilation in amyotrophic lateral sclerosis. *Eur Neurol*, 2008, 59, 164–171.

[50] Volanti, P; Cibella, F; Sarva, M. Predictors of non-invasive ventilation tolerance in amyotrophic lateral sclerosis. *J Neurol Sci*, 2011, 303, 114–118.

[51] Jackson, CE; Gronseth, G; Rosenfeld, J. Randomized double-blind study of botulinum toxin type B for sialorrhea in ALS patients. *Muscle Nerve*, 2009, 39, 137–143

[52] Winck, JC; Goncalves, MR; Lourenco, C. Effects of mechanical insufflation-exsufflation on respiratory parameters for patients with chronic airway secretion encumbrance. *Chest*, 2004, 126, 774–780.

[53] Chatwin, M; Toussaint, M; Goncalves, MR. Airway clearance techniques in neuromuscular disorders: a state of the art review. *Respir Med*, 2018, 136, 98–110

[54] Sancho, J; Servera, E; Diaz, J. Efficacy of mechanical insufflation-exsufflation in medically stable patients with amyotrophic lateral sclerosis. *Chest*, 2004, 125, 1400–1405.

[55] Rafiq, MK; Bradburn, M; Proctor, AR. A preliminary randomized trial of the mechanical insufflator-exsufflator versus breath-stacking technique in patients with amyotrophic lateral sclerosis. *Amyotroph Lateral Scler Frontotemporal Degener*, 2015, 16, 448–455.

[56] Toussaint, M; Boitano, LJ; Gathot, V. Limits of effective cough-augmentation techniques in patients with neuromuscular disease. *Respir Care*, 2009, 54, 359–366.

[57] Trebbia, G; Lacombe, M; Fermanian, C. Cough determinants in patients with neuromuscular disease. *Respir Physiol Neurobiol*, 2005, 146, 291–300.

[58] Fiorentino, G; Annunziata, A; Gaeta, AM; Lanza, M; Esquinas, A. Continuous noninvasive ventilation for respiratory failure in patients with amyotrophic lateral sclerosis: current perspectives. *Degener Neurol Neuromuscul Dis.*, 2018, 8, 55-61. Published 2018 Sep 4.

[59] Vianello, A; Arcaro, G; Palmieri, A; Ermani, M; Braccioni, F; Gallan, F; Soraru', G; Pegoraro, E. Survival and quality of life after tracheostomy for acute respiratory failure in patients with amyotrophic lateral sclerosis. *J. Crit. Care*, 2011, 26, 329. e7–14.

[60] Tagami, M; Kimura, F; Nakajima, H; Ishida, S; Fujiwara, S; Doi, Y; Hosokawa, T; Yamane, K; Unoda, K; Hirose, T; et al. Tracheostomy and invasive ventilation in Japanese ALS patients: decision-making and survival analysis: 1990-2010. *J. Neurol. Sci.*, 2014, 344, 158–64.

[61] Hirose, T; Kimura, F; Tani, H. Clinical characteristics of long-term survival with non-invasive ventilation and factors affecting the

transition to invasive ventilation in ALS. *Muscle Nerve*, 2018, 58, 770–776.

[62] Spataro, R; Bono, V; Marchese, S. Tracheostomy mechanical ventilation in patients with amyotrophic lateral sclerosis: clinical features and survival analysis. *J Neurol Sci*, 2012, 323, 66–70.

[63] Andersen, PM; Kuzma-Kozakiewicz, M; Keller, J. Therapeutic decisions in ALS patients: cross-cultural differences and clinical implications. *J Neurol*, 2018, 265, 1600–1606.

[64] Aho-Ozhan, HE; Bohm, S; Keller, J. Experience matters: neurologists' perspectives on ALS patients' well-being. *J Neurol*, 2017, 264, 639–646.

[65] Markovic, N; Povitz, M; Smith, J. Patterns of non-invasive ventilation in amyotrophic lateral sclerosis. *Can J Neurol Sci*, 2018, 6, 1–6.

[66] Ganzini, L; Johnston, WS; Silveira, MJ. The final month of life in patients with ALS. *Neurology*, 2002, 59, 428–31.

[67] Kettemann, D; Funke, A; Maier, A. Clinical characteristics and course of dying in patients with amyotrophic lateral sclerosis withdrawing from long-term ventilation. *Amyotroph Lateral Scler Frontotemporal Degener*, 2017, 18, 53–59.

INDEX

#

3D images, 31

A

absorption spectra, 25
action potential, 129, 130, 145, 151
adult stem cells, 6
afferent nerve fiber, 25
age, 19, 35, 71, 78, 108, 113
aggregation, 4, 5, 9, 12, 13, 17, 32, 33, 34, 60, 70, 75, 81, 85, 89
alters, 157
amino, 13
amplitude, 44, 129
animal models, viii, 2, 21, 26, 39, 46, 55, 57, 92
anisotropy, 46, 47, 48, 58
anomalous diffusion, 53, 54, 70, 76, 94
antibody, 25, 42, 136
anticholinergic, 167, 168
antioxidant, 5, 79
antisense RNA, 13, 35

arterial blood gas, 158, 160
astrocytes, 13, 18, 32, 36, 41, 60, 87, 89
astrogliosis, 4, 12, 19, 21, 36
asymptomatic, 160, 172
atrophy, 12, 18, 32, 41, 126, 145
autobiographical memory, 114
axonal degeneration, 19, 68, 69, 70, 94
axonal pathology, 69, 93
axons, 10, 11, 17, 18, 21, 22, 25, 38, 55, 69, 149, 150

B

biomarkers, vii, x, 20, 32, 37, 38, 54, 85, 88, 89, 125
biopsy, 130, 131, 133, 134, 135, 136, 138, 139, 141, 147
body weight, 16, 162
borderline personality disorder, 118
brain, 7, 9, 23, 31, 33, 35, 36, 45, 51, 57, 59, 71, 77, 79, 80, 84, 86, 88, 89, 126, 130, 140, 147
brain stem, 19, 50, 126
brain structure, 36
breathing, 101, 108, 156, 158, 162

C

cachexia, 128
carbon dioxide (CO$_2$), 133, 155, 158, 171
caregivers, 111, 121, 168, 169
CBC, 93
CD8+, 32, 36
CDM, 18
cDNA, 9, 34
cell biology, 29, 73
cell body, 25, 37
cell culture, 7, 81
cell death, 9, 12, 13, 20, 41
cell line, 4, 7
central nervous system (CNS), 18, 28, 29, 35, 36, 46, 49, 50, 52, 71, 132
cerebral cortex, 27
cerebrospinal fluid, 51
clinical application, 68, 162
clinical symptoms, 162
clinical trials, 70, 87
coefficient of variation, 133
cognitive deficits, 111
cognitive function, 173
cognitive impairment, x, 112, 155, 167
cognitive performance, x, 155, 157
communicative intent, 111
complexity, 3, 4, 5, 7, 9, 10, 18, 28, 44, 52, 53, 54, 56, 77, 114, 163
compulsion, 119, 120
conduction, 128, 129, 130, 135, 143, 144, 145, 154
contextualization, ix, 100, 109, 113
corpus callosum, 46, 59
cortex, 10, 15, 18, 27, 39, 50, 67, 86, 115, 127, 128, 132, 140, 148
cortical neurons, 138
cough, xi, 156, 167, 168, 179
cytoplasm, 6, 15, 16, 23, 33, 37, 39, 41
cytoskeleton, 32, 38
cytotoxicity, 6, 33, 73

D

defects, 5, 12, 17, 19, 32, 38, 44, 91
deficiency, 18, 74, 170
deficit, xi, 133, 137, 156, 168
dementia, 8, 90, 149
demyelination, 19, 55, 67, 87, 90
dendrites, 13, 16, 22, 23, 25, 40
dendritic spines, 39
denervation, v, x, 12, 13, 17, 18, 19, 32, 41, 42, 125, 127, 129, 131, 134, 141
depression, x, 2, 102, 117, 155, 170
detection, 5, 19, 30, 33, 43, 76, 94, 134, 137, 139, 149, 158, 160
diaphragm, 42, 158, 165, 174
disability, 127, 133, 161, 170
disease progression, 13, 17, 18, 31, 55, 71, 77, 87, 160
diseases, viii, ix, 2, 7, 10, 22, 59, 90, 92, 95, 100, 101, 104, 107, 110, 126, 141, 165
Drosophila, 8, 60, 64, 71, 74, 75, 83, 85, 91
drug addiction, 111
drug targets, 85
drug testing, 3
drugs, 14, 36, 166, 167, 168
dysphagia, 133
dyspnea, 156, 160, 170

E

electrocardiogram (ECG), 133
electron(s), 24, 39
emotion regulation, 102, 113
emotional experience, 122
emotional state, 103
encoding, 11, 12, 13, 20, 89
endonuclease, 9
endoscopy, 133
energy expenditure, 157
eukaryotic cell, 5

Index

evoked potential, 129, 130, 135, 140, 142, 143, 145, 146, 148, 150, 152, 153
experimental autoimmune encephalomyelitis, 90

F

false negative, 127
false positive, 127, 143
fluorescence, 21, 22, 23, 24, 27, 29, 33, 34, 54, 70, 86
fluorophores, 29, 31, 78
forebrain, 35, 40
frontal cortex, 126

G

ganglion, 81
gender effects, 71
gene expression, 15, 65, 151
general anaesthesia, 166
genes, 2, 5, 8, 18
genetic background, 14, 77
genetic mutations, viii, 2, 15, 55, 57
genetics, viii, 2, 8, 83
genitourinary tract, 105
genome, 5
glia, 25, 37, 81
glucose tolerance, 133
glucoside, 13
glutamate, 4, 12
glycoproteins, 71
gray matter, 15, 73, 144

H

Hawking, Stephen, 169
health services, 112
heart failure, 105
heart rate, 133, 134, 150

hippocampus, 18, 28, 33, 37, 50, 53, 127
hopelessness, 102, 112, 114, 121
hospitalization, 108, 171

I

idiopathic pulmonary hypertension, ix, 100, 104
illness experience, v, vii, ix, 99, 100, 101, 102, 104, 107, 111, 112, 113
imagery, ix, 100, 103, 106, 107, 110
images, 30, 31, 38, 42, 43
imaging modalities, 57
imaging systems, 31
immunohistochemistry, 31, 40
impairments, ix, 100, 101
in vitro, viii, 2, 3, 7, 26, 32
in vivo, viii, 2, 3, 26, 45, 49, 50, 55, 57, 91, 93
ion channels, 95, 96
ipsilateral, 105

L

labeling, 23, 25, 26
laryngoscopy, 163, 177
larynx, 133, 137
lateral sclerosis, vii, 2, 40, 67, 101, 115, 119, 126, 130, 142, 145, 146, 147, 148, 152, 173, 175
lipoproteins, 37
living conditions, x, 156
localization, 5, 13, 24, 25, 30, 31, 32, 33, 34, 35, 36, 38, 39, 41, 70, 76
locomotor, 8, 9, 11, 13, 16, 66, 89
lupus, 18, 122
lymphocytes, 36

M

macrophages, 35
magnetic field, viii, 2, 43, 45, 50
magnetic resonance imaging (MRI), vii, viii, 1, 2, 43, 44, 45, 46, 51, 53, 54, 56, 57, 59, 61, 62, 65, 67, 69, 73, 76, 79, 82, 86, 90, 93, 94, 95, 96, 97, 140, 147, 148
malnutrition, xi, 156
MBP, 32, 37, 56
MCP, 36
MCP-1, 36
mechanical ventilation, 177, 180
medicine, viii, ix, 51, 99, 100, 101, 104, 114, 115
mellitus, 142
memory, 83, 114, 120
mesenchymal stem cells, 78, 86
meta-analysis, 63
metabolism, 4, 9, 15, 91
methodology, 16, 123
microRNA, 20, 35, 61
microscopy, 21, 22, 23, 29, 30, 31, 32, 33, 34, 35, 39, 54, 60, 65, 76, 79, 86, 133, 136, 144
models, viii, 1, 2, 3, 4, 5, 7, 8, 10, 11, 12, 13, 15, 16, 17, 18, 20, 21, 22, 26, 27, 32, 34, 35, 36, 37, 39, 40, 41, 43, 44, 46, 49, 50, 51, 52, 53, 54, 55, 57, 59, 62, 65, 66, 70, 72, 79, 80, 82, 84, 87, 88, 91, 93, 96, 165
morphology, 17, 27, 40, 51, 52, 81
morphometric, 23, 24
motor neuron disease, vii, x, 66, 72, 82, 121, 125, 141, 142, 143, 146, 175
motor neurons, 4, 6, 10, 11, 12, 16, 17, 18, 19, 20, 27, 32, 33, 34, 38, 39, 40, 41, 42, 63, 64, 68, 70, 72, 85, 101, 126, 127, 137, 141
MRI diffusion, 2, 43, 46, 51, 54, 55, 56, 57, 94

mRNA, 25, 27
multiple sclerosis, 85
muscle atrophy, 12, 17, 19
muscles, vii, x, 19, 20, 42, 126, 151, 155, 157, 160, 164
musculoskeletal, 138
mutant, 5, 8, 11, 12, 13, 16, 18, 19, 33, 34, 39, 41, 63, 74, 75, 78, 80, 86, 87, 89
mutant proteins, 5, 39
mutation(s), 2, 5, 6, 7, 8, 9, 10, 11, 12, 13, 14, 17, 18, 19, 27, 34, 38, 39, 41, 42, 66, 80, 81, 91, 142, 148
myelin, 37, 55
myopathy, 19, 64
myosin, 24

N

narrative medicine, viii, 99, 101, 104, 116
nerve, 20, 23, 42, 128, 129, 130, 131, 133, 134, 135, 136, 137, 139, 140, 142, 143, 144, 145, 146, 147, 148, 150, 151, 154, 173
nerve biopsy, 139
nerve fibers, 142, 143, 147
nervous system, 8, 18, 25, 27
neural function, 152
neural network, 15
neurobiology, 26
neuroblastoma, 4
neurodegeneration, 4, 7, 9, 21, 31, 59, 70, 71, 75, 82, 87, 90, 91, 131, 136
neurodegenerative diseases, viii, 2, 3, 4, 5, 7, 9, 21, 22, 26, 27, 54, 62, 65, 84, 90
neurodegenerative disorders, 9, 58, 66, 72
neurofibrillary tangles, 13, 16
neurofilaments, 34, 38, 42, 87
neuroimaging, v, vii, viii, 1, 2, 3, 57, 64, 84, 88, 92, 148, 149
neuroinflammation, 13, 16, 32, 36, 63, 80, 85, 86

neurological disability, 85
neuronal circuits, 22
neurons, 4, 7, 8, 12, 13, 16, 17, 18, 20, 22, 23, 26, 27, 31, 33, 34, 35, 39, 40, 41, 59, 67, 70, 81, 87, 89, 126, 137, 144, 149
neuropathic pain, 136, 138, 142
neuropathy, 128, 144, 145, 146, 147, 152
neurophysiology, 146
neuroprotection, 30
neuroscience, 26, 30, 31, 51, 62, 73, 78, 81, 86
neurotoxicity, 60, 75, 85
non-invasive ventilation (NIV), v, x, 155, 156, 157, 159, 161, 162, 163, 164, 165, 166, 167, 168, 170, 171, 173, 174, 175, 176, 177, 178, 179, 180
norepinephrine, 133, 151
Nrf2, 79
nucleic acid, 23, 25
nucleolus, 41
nucleotide sequence, 68
nucleus, 15, 20, 39, 44, 50, 126

O

obstruction, 160, 161, 163, 176, 177
obstructive lung disease, 162
oligodendrocytes, 33, 37, 41, 55, 73, 126
opioids, 170
optical microscopy, viii, 2, 21, 22, 56, 68
optical systems, 31
organism, 3, 4, 5, 7
organs, 132, 136
orthopnea, 160
orthostatic intolerance, 133
oxidative stress, 13, 17, 34, 60

P

pain, 136, 137, 138, 139, 151, 170
palliative, xi, 156, 170

panic attack, 167
paralysis, 2, 16, 18, 41, 126, 169
Parkinsonism, 90
participants, ix, 100, 104, 106, 107, 108, 113
pathogenesis, 6, 35, 74, 93, 126
pathology, 4, 5, 7, 9, 16, 20, 33, 43, 46, 69, 74, 91, 93, 129, 142, 145, 147, 148
pathophysiological, 3
pathophysiology, 6, 21, 57
pathways, 3, 4, 5, 9, 10, 36, 67, 79, 136, 140, 143
pectoralis major, 105
peripheral blood, 133
peripheral nervous system, 127, 128
pharmacotherapy, 118
phenotype(s), 7, 9, 13, 15, 16, 17, 19, 20, 31, 71, 72, 84, 86, 143, 158
phosphorylation, 17, 32
photobleaching, 26
photons, 24
physical health, 114, 115, 118
pneumonia, 162, 171
point mutation, 12, 17
positive end expiratory pressure, 176
prefrontal cortex, 28, 40, 126
premature death, 12
progenitor cells, 37
prognosis, xi, 2, 54, 145, 156, 166, 168, 172
protein misfolding, 5, 65
protein-protein interactions, 5, 6, 33
proteins, 4, 5, 8, 15, 16, 17, 21, 24, 25, 29, 32, 35, 36, 38, 39, 52, 55, 63, 64, 75, 78, 83, 85, 89, 97, 126
proteoglycans, 52
protons, 44, 96
psychological distress, 102
psychology, 115, 122
psychometric properties, 121
psychotherapy, 103, 121, 122
pulmonary hypertension, 105

Q

qualitative research, 113, 117, 122
quality of life, viii, x, 99, 101, 102, 116, 155, 156, 157, 159, 162, 168, 169, 171, 173, 175, 179
quality of life (QoL), viii, x, 99, 101, 102, 116, 120, 121, 155, 156, 157, 159, 162, 165, 168, 169, 171, 173, 175, 179
quantum dots, 26, 83

R

radiation, 167, 178
radiation therapy, 167
radiculopathy, 129
radiotherapy, 166
reaction time, 144
recalling, 108
receptor(s), 19, 32, 43, 133, 151, 168
recognition, 24, 79, 103
referential activity, ix, 100, 101, 102, 109, 115, 118
reflexes, 130, 144
regeneration, 39, 73, 135, 143
regression, 67
rehabilitation, 120
relatives, 120
relaxation, 44, 80
remyelination, 67, 87
respiratory failure, vii, x, 155, 168, 179
response, 5, 11, 126, 133, 149, 173
reverse transcriptase, 9
rhinitis, 165
RNA, 4, 5, 9, 12, 13, 15, 16, 23, 25, 32, 35, 62, 66, 79, 91
RNA processing, 6, 12, 35

S

salivary gland, 166, 167
salivary glands, 167
schizophrenia, 58
self-identity, ix, 100, 101, 113
sensitivity, 24, 43, 44, 51, 86, 158, 160
sensitization, 138
sensory, v, vii, ix, x, 70, 100, 103, 105, 107, 110, 125, 127, 128, 129, 130, 131, 132, 133, 135, 137, 138, 139, 140, 141, 142, 144, 145, 146, 148, 149, 150, 151, 152, 154
sensory experience, 103, 111
sensory symptoms, 135
sensory system, 150
signal-to-noise ratio, 26
signs, 17, 19, 126, 130, 135, 137, 159, 161
skeletal muscle, 18, 19, 41
skin, 132, 133, 134, 135, 136, 138, 139, 140, 141, 142, 146, 147, 151, 165
sleep apnea, 160, 172
sleep disorders, 172
SNAP, 129, 130, 135
sniff nasal inspiratory pressure (SNIP), 156, 158, 160
social cognition, 115
social construct, 116
social desirability, 113
social psychology, 118
social support, 113, 122
somatomotor, 126
spasticity, 40, 101
specialists, 160, 169, 170
species, 20, 25, 87
speech, 108, 157, 164
spinal cord, 4, 10, 11, 15, 19, 20, 28, 29, 32, 33, 34, 35, 36, 37, 39, 40, 41, 42, 47, 48, 55, 65, 68, 69, 74, 76, 80, 81, 82, 89, 140, 142
spine, 12, 13, 15, 16, 24, 39, 67, 126

stability, 27
stabilization, 38
stem cell lines, 60
stem cells, 6, 7, 37, 61, 83
stimulation, 148
stimulus, 133, 139
stress, 5, 9, 34, 75, 86, 118, 134
stress granules, 34, 75
stress response, 5
structure, 12, 18, 27, 30, 43, 44, 45, 52, 53, 55, 56, 67, 119
survival, x, 14, 17, 31, 71, 76, 86, 127, 155, 157, 159, 160, 162, 164, 166, 168, 169, 171, 173, 174, 175, 176, 178, 179, 180
survival rate, 173
swelling, 23, 61, 135
sympathetic nervous system, 150
symptoms, x, 14, 15, 16, 18, 66, 73, 101, 102, 105, 118, 126, 133, 135, 137, 155, 159, 166, 170
synapse, 16, 42, 74
synaptic transmission, 58
synaptic vesicles, 8
syndrome, ix, 100, 104, 169, 171
synthesis, 37, 119

T

temporal lobe, 127
text analysis, 101, 106, 119
text mining, 116
therapeutic approaches, 3
therapeutic effect, 6
therapeutic interventions, 170
therapeutic targets, 3, 4
therapeutics, 21, 57
therapy, 6, 7, 77, 86, 156, 159, 167, 168, 170, 178

tibialis anterior, 42
toxicity, 5, 9, 13, 33, 66, 75, 80, 85
tracheostomy, 156, 169, 179
traumatic brain injury, 68
traumatic experiences, 103
treatment, viii, x, 2, 6, 14, 21, 27, 36, 65, 78, 101, 114, 115, 144, 155, 156, 157, 161, 166, 170, 176, 178

U

ubiquitin, 4, 12, 13, 27, 32, 35, 126, 149
upper airways, vii, x, 155, 168

V

valsalva, 133
ventilation, x, 119, 155, 156, 159, 161, 162, 164, 165, 166, 168, 169, 170, 172, 173, 174, 175, 176, 177, 178, 179, 180
vesicle, 12, 17, 39
vessels, 133
vibration, 130, 137
visualization, 22, 23, 27
vital capacity (VC), 133, 156, 158, 160, 178

W

weakness, 126, 132, 137, 157, 170
well-being, 116, 118, 180

Y

yeast, 5, 33, 73, 75, 83, 85, 90